HUNTSVILLE

HUNTSVILLE
A LEE W. HICKOK NOVEL

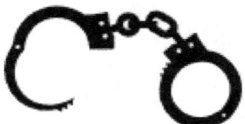

William Lynes, MD

Huntsville
March 2018
First Edition
ISBN# 13: 978-1986549134
Copyright Pending

William Lynes, MD Books
Lynesonline.com

Bible quotations from "New International Version." Copyright 1973, 1978, 1984 Zondervan Corp.

Dr. Seuss quotations from "The Cat in the Hat" Copyright 1957

Mark Twain quotations from "Adventures of Huckleberry Finn" Copyright 1884

All rights are reserved solely by the author who certifies that all contents are original and do not infringe on any other person or work. No portion of this book may be reproduced without written permission of the author. All names of persons are fictitious and any resemblance to real persons is purely coincidental. Real names of places are used to set locale, but the specific sites and events described herein are purely fictitious.

Icon made by Freepik from www.flaticon.com

ACKNOWLEDGEMENT

I dedicate this book to my family, Patrice, Christopher, Alexander and Nicholas Lynes. Thank you for your love and support.

Chapter 1

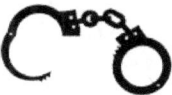

The moonless sky was steamy, sweltering dust rising in the air after the intense heat of the day. Gravel cracked as the rusty Malibu turned into *THirsty THirties*, the Friday night just beginning. An angry man exited the vehicle to the jukebox of a worn-out Texas beer saloon, as his cowboy boots crunched on the crushed rock.

Within the bar was a small disinterested crowd playing pool and drinking cold brew. The angry man stood in the doorway, wondering about his night, thinking about mayhem. He was tallish, stick-thin with a light black complexion, steel blue menacing eyes, and a mouthful of golden tines. His hair was organized into black nappy cornrows which hung to his shoulders. A wife-beater shirt covered his chest, where a typical tattoo green eagle chest ink peeked out through the armholes.

Their eyes locked a daring sexual signal, a white bleached blond girl tending bar with a swollen curvy chest covered by a sleeveless pink top worn over tight denim jeans.

The angry man, Billie James Sampson, took a seat at the rotting bar, demanding a *Bud* but wanting much more. She served the man quickly, the ice-cold bottle set on a white paper napkin which said just **TH--TH** in red. The music blared a stifling overhead beat, Donna Summer's *She Works Hard for the Money* serenading the barmaid who left without luck looking for a smoke.

He followed the woman into the lot, picking her up under a sole bug covered pole light. She was interested, knowing the man from before. A romp in the Malibu sealed her fate. She wasn't one for rough, however, and tried to leave, the doors locked before her exit. He beat her for not caring, her overly made up face a mess as he pushed her out the now open door to the gravel below. She was disrespectful to the man, a baseball bat correcting her mistake. Her bloody face and twisted dead body were left behind, the Malibu crushing her golden ringed left hand as it exited.

Statement, deposition, testimony and appeal followed the facts always the same. He preyed on her, following her out to the car. A bat was ready, premeditating his actions. A history of violence and the brutal nature involving rape landed him First Degree Murder with Special Circumstances. The red-bricked *Walls* section of Huntsville Texas Department of Corrections Death Row was his intended home for the next eight years, waiting for the needle to end his misery.

The pain frequently appeared during his entire adult life, a horrible discomfort that came and went in his flank and groin. It was why he was so angry, many said. He heard that so often that he came to believe and rely on the fact. His first day on the row was met with an episode so bad that the disbelieving staff eventually put him in the medical ward. He came to realize, however, that medical was not better than a cell. Oh, maybe a gurney with an elevatable head, a supply of towels, and a gray metal bucket to puke in. Beyond that, you were on your own except for one fact.

Bobbie was a black veteran-medic of the Vietnam war. He was a massive man with huge pectoral peaks giving rise to the name behind his back: *Boobie*. As a member of the healthcare industry, he wasn't committed, the man had the sympathy of a rock. He ran the unit, however, and his impression was law.

The only key to the medicine case was his, hanging like a chandelier between his lofty precipices. And with it came that golden fluid of mercy, morphine. You had to be double-dog sick to receive a dose. Nausea helped fever as well, fractures with exposed bone, borderline. What really impressed Bobbie however, was vomiting, especially projectile, but only after one bucket was produced.

"I's hurting Bobbie. Bobbie where are ya man!" This went on nearly all night with the only response being: "I'll get to you, Sampson." Only when he vomited a full bucket was the action prompt, meaning within the hour.

"You'se really hurting Sampson?"

"I pray on my dead Mother's grave," Sampson said spitting. "I ain't spoofing no way, Bobbie please I know I brave, but I needs the needle."

Bobbie eventually made it to his bedside. Two other inmates occupied the ward, neither seeming to be requiring much of his time. He lifted Sampson's puke bucket, impressed by its weight. He shook his head and placed a hand on the man's forehead. "Wow, you a little warm." Out of his white coat pocket, he pulled a morphine sulfate ampule and injected 10 mg intramuscularly.

Sampson's fate was two days of continuing pain with control at the whim of Bobbie.

"The stone is down there Bobbie, I feel like I need to pee all the time." Here Sampson's feeling the need to void suggested that the stone was in the lowermost or distal ureter, that part of the tube from the kidney to the bladder that travels in the wall of the bladder. A stone here inflames the bladder and gives this feeling.

"Well yaw-all's been here two full days Sampson, and not any better. Doctor McCormick will see you and make a deposition."

Two days later, still in pain, he was transferred.

Doctor James "Slim" McCormack was a 65-year-old general surgeon who practiced for 35 years at Conroe Regional Medical Center in Conroe Texas, a 30-minute ride south on Highway 45. His long surgical history at the medical center gave his OR privileges grandfather status including all urologic procedures.

He was tall and despite his nickname, had a brooding paunch, with a balding red-brown tonsured head, blue eyes covered with thick black spectacles. He was dressed as always in surgical scrubs, a dirty white coat jammed with paper slips, odds, and ends, and wore paper-shoe covered boots. He met his new patient on the surgical ward of Conroe Regional, the door flanked by two dark gray uniformed, hatted, and armed corrections officers sitting across from one another in gray metal folding chairs.

"I like your tie clasps," Slim said to both officers, each having handcuff shaped clasps over black issued ties, one wearing dense black sunglasses. Neither said anything, but both shook their heads and smiled narrow smiles. Slim grabbed the clipboard hanging from the door and took a moment to eye the vital signs.

"Mr. Sampson, Doctor McCormack." Not bothering to shake the man's hand he stood at the foot of the bed. "I understand you've got a stone."

Sampson sat the head of his bed up and said nothing. He had the type of face that belied anger at every turn, his golden tines shining through a severe scowl that said: *who the Hell are you?*

Slim moved to the side of the bed and asked. "Where yaw-all hurting?"

With reluctance, Sampson placed his hand on his left flank and then pointed as well to his left groin.

Slim moved to the x-ray box on the wall next to the bed. He grabbed an x-ray jacket and slid up several films. He took his pen from his white coat and pointed to a white round density in the pelvis. "This here is your stone. It's about 7 millimeters and in the left ureter by the bladder. Yaw-all having a hard time urinating?"

Sampson just shook his head, yes, his light blue eyes staring without emotion at the man, his facies revealing a sincere desire to kill the Doctor.

"Mr. Sampson, can I call you Billie?" He turned from the view-box to the patient.

Sampson just glared and shook his head negatively.

"Well…okay yaw-all. I plan to make an incision here." Slim moved to the patient's left side and traced out an incision in the left pelvis. "Yaw-all will have tubes. It will hurt some, then yaw-all be okay. Got any questions?"

"When does I get to eat?"

"Right after the operation, yaw-all have to drink liquids first."

"I needs my *kicker!*"

Slim grimaced. "Kicker?" He turned to the officers at the door with a question on his face.

"Dude…bitch mint…Morph!"

Slim seemed to understand the last phrase. "Oh, certainly we'll dose you until your pain's gone."

Sampson smiled a tiny smile, closed his eyes, and electrically lowered the head of his bed.

It was left sided, usually, but it had occurred on the right before. He was a poor Texas black man with no health care and so never sought out a physician. Within 18 months after surgery, three separate left-sided episodes and similar surgeries were performed and then it was back again, severe left sided flank pain radiating to the left groin, with nausea and vomiting.

If there was one thing positive about Huntsville it was access, too often poor, but access to medical care. Recurrent left-sided kidney stone was the diagnosis, Slim was frustrated, and quickly the solution was to remove that kidney. When one month post-operatively a right-sided episode occurred, Mr. Sampson was in trouble.

Stones are formed in the kidney. When they drop out and obstruct the urine flow in the ureter, the tube from the kidney to the bladder, the most prominent symptom is severe pain or renal colic, usually beginning in the flank over the kidney and radiating to the groin.

With two kidneys, the obstruction of one is metabolically insignificant, the other kidney can do the function of two, that is filter the blood of toxins. In Mr. Sampson's case, he now had a solitary right kidney. Obstruction of that single renal unit, in addition to pain, results more importantly in the absence of urine production, and acute renal or kidney failure, a medical emergency.

Sampson was well until sudden pain caused him to jump from the small corner mounted metal cot collapsing on the floor. It was not supposed to happen, his left kidney removed to treat the recurrent episodes of left renal colic. It was unmistakable, however, renal colic pain, nothing in the world like it to someone who had experienced it before. But the pain was right sided, and so the saga began.

"Hey, Boss, get the F*** down here, I's hurting," he yelled down the hall rapping his metal cup on the bars of his Wall's unit Huntsville cell.

The guard walked slowly, stopping in front of Sampson. He said nothing.

"I's hurt," he said with a hand on his right flank. He put his hand over his mouth stopping an emesis for the moment. "I's need to go to medical," he said now seemingly out of breath.

When Bobbie saw him and the empty urinal he did something he did only rarely. He took the immediate initiative to get a doctor to see the man in medical. He bypassed Slim McCormack, being frustrated himself with the zip-zip course of surgeries and now an obstructed right kidney.

Doctor J.D. Wilson was an internist who practiced and was locally trained at the Sam Houston Medical center. He was perhaps the best medical doctor that Sampson had ever encountered.

"Mr. Sampson, I am Doctor Wilson. I am an internist at Sam Houston."

Sampson said nothing. He lay on his left side, his eyes closed, breathing heavily. Wilson performed a physical exam finding an elevation of blood pressure, pulse, and respiratory rate. His weight was up five kilograms from fluid retention. His legs showed pitting edema. He had *candy texture* lips, graying dry skin, and pronounced deep tendon reflexes with a percussion hammer. In addition, he had bilateral nystagmus, a condition where the eyes rapidly beat laterally when deviated. The exam was consistent with renal failure.

Wilson asked Bobbie to draw a series of blood tests and obtain a KUB, a kidney ureter and bladder single-shot x-ray of the abdomen. He then moved to the gray metal desk in the center of the medic ward to write a note.

The water pitcher on the bedside table fell to the ground after an abortive grab by Sampson. He yelled an incomprehensible yell.

The man put his head and back in extension and began a generalized tonic-clonic seizure. Wilson jumped up, knocking his chart off the desk and ran to the patient's side.

"He's having a seizure, Bobbie," Wilson said as he slid to his back on the wet floor. "Crap." He grabbed the rail of the bed and pulled himself upright. He reached to the wall retrieving a plastic mouth guard which he forced into Sampson's mouth protecting the patient's tongue from violent biting. Oxygen by nasal cannula was placed, the volume turned to maximum, the man kept on his side. "Ten milligrams of diazepam IV Bobbie, hook him up to an EKG. Let's load him with 50mg over a minute of phenytoin," a powerful anti-seizure medicine. Wilson took just a moment to straighten the back of his soaked white coat and retrieve his stethoscope from the floor.

Bobbie was running getting drugs, hooking up the bedside EKG, and infusing medication. Sampson was breathing heavily and sweating. Within minutes of the diazepam, the patient began to quiet. His shaking began to slow and he snored loudly in a rhythmic manner, drool collecting on the mouth guard.

Bobbie returned and tossed some paper labs on the gurney. "Here's his labs, Doc. Do you still want that phenytoin?"

"Crap," Wilson said again after reviewing the labs. "His uric acid level is 15 and his potassium is 5.9." He looked up at the nurse. "This guy's in trouble, renal failure, put in a Foley." Here he referred to a catheter in the bladder held in place with a small balloon.

"The phenytoin, do you still want it?"

"Yes, but make sure it goes in slowly, say over five minutes now that I see these labs. We need a 12 lead EKG stat, Bobbie! Let's give him an amp of calcium, an amp of D50 glucose, a half amp of insulin, and an amp of bicarb."

"Orders, doctor! I need written orders." Bobbie opened a catheter tray, pulled the man's pants down and began placing the Foley. "There is no urine in the bladder." A patient down the room began yelling for pain medicine. "Cut it Michaels yaw-all have to wait!"

"Do that EKG, I'll get the chart and start writing. I'll call x-ray in here for that KUB." Wilson moved and picked up the patient chart off the floor. He made a quick call to x-ray. He then returned to the bedside. The chart had sprung open. At first, he began to straighten it, but then, reflecting on the emergency of the situation, stopped. He found an empty order sheet and began writing. The glucose, insulin, and bicarbonate were to force potassium back into the cell reducing the potassium level in the blood. The calcium stabilized the heart to the effects of potassium.

"Here is the 12 lead, I haven't marked it yet." The tracing was a long single column EKG done on an old machine with leads held to the patient with suction cups. The twelve leads followed each other down the narrow tracing. Wilson quickly marked each lead with a pen, then perused the tracing. "He has some QRS widening Bobbie, from the hyperkalemia." Here he referred to an EKG change consistent with the elevated potassium.

X-ray arrived, positioned the man on his back and slid a pillow-case covered x-ray cassette under him. Bobbie and Wilson moved across the room and the film was exposed.

The KUB arrived and was placed upon the x-ray view box. Doctor Wilson took time from his orders to view the film.

There was an obvious seven to eight-millimeter density overlying the mid-right ureter with several small calcifications in the area of the kidney. No kidney outline was visible on the left. Wilson stared at the film, then walked to Sampson's bed. He uncovered his flank first on the right and then to reveal the left well-healed incisions. He turned to Bobbie and spoke really to himself. "Why does this man not have a left kidney? Now he has an obstructed right kidney, with acute renal failure and seizures. Why? Bobbie, why?"

"Kidney stones," was the answer.

Chapter 2

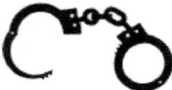

It was midnight in October and the annual departmental party was in full swing for 1985 when the chief of urology at the University of Texas Medical Branch in Galveston Texas (UTMB) stood to address the crowd.

"Let me get your attention." He said, tapping a small spoon on the edge of a fresh Manhattan after consuming the maraschino cherry. Fuad Fadi, MD stood in the great-room of the Lee W. Hickok's restored Victorian home trying to be heard over the talk that dominated the room. "I have an announcement," he said as everyone quieted down and took a seat. Doctor Fadi was a distinguished middle-eastern man with slightly receding brown hair sprinkled with distinguished gray highlights and a similarly colored bushy brown mustache. He was dressed in a black and white tuxedo and a silly paper hat.

"Thank you, group. As you know, I am old. I am really old"

There was laughing in the room and cries of "no Fuad." "Fuad for President!"

"Yes, my wife tells me this so often." He turned to a beautiful brown-haired woman dressed in a white cocktail dress and embraced her. Holding her hand now he went on. "I am now old and have decided to step down from my administrative chores appointing Doctor Lee W. Hickok as departmental chief."

"Lee W…. Lee W….," followed from the crowd.

"Well, I see this is a popular decision." Fadi paused and took in the light-hearted atmosphere. "I have been at the university now for twenty years, the chief for seven of those. I remember Lee W. as a medical student, intern, resident, chief resident, and now urologic attending and find him to be overly qualified for this position of chief."

There were laughs all around.

"All kidding aside, Lee W. is a talented urologist, doctor, and an honorable man. Lee W. I give you the floor."

Lee W. approached the man. What began as a handshake between colleagues became a heartfelt embrace. Lee W. was a tallish man with a full head of dark-brown hair tinged in the temples with gray. He too wore a tuxedo, black with a black shirt and white bow-tie. Unlike much of the crowd, he wore shiny black cowboy boots, somewhat of a personal declaration to the state of Texas. Lee W. held up his sparkling mineral water with a lemon twist and nodded to the man moving to the center of the room. He was an alcoholic, now sober for 47 and ½ months. His sobriety really began with the tragic post-operative death of the Governor of Texas, J.T. Splinter, an extramarital affair and death of a young medical student; his alcoholism and infidelity resulting in separation. Not that the desire was not there, he had several prolific dreams about drinking in the days leading up to the party, and he still kept empty bottles of Jim Beam or Sweet Amber at strategic locations to reinforce himself with a sniff.

The invitees all stood and shook hands with Lee W who returned them and made a point to embrace his reconciled loving wife, Amber. There were laughing and sincere compliments to a man who was respected by all. Then the phone rang.

Lee W. looked at Amber, thinking the worst. Yes, he was technically on call, but a call from the hospital would go through the residents in the room. Everyone stood looking at him after eyeing their empty pagers. Lee W. moved to his office anxious to use his new space phone, wondering the origin of the call.

"Lee W., its Abbott Frankenstein." Doctor Frankenstein was the president of the university, a call from him now was entirely out of the ordinary. He was a political force at the university, and some said the next in line for a state senate position in Austin.

"Abbott, nice of you to call. What can I do for you?"

"Well, I am sorry to interrupt your festivities. I understand that tonight is your departmental dinner party?"

Lee W. thought to himself that the phone call must have been to congratulate him. He was somewhat relieved when Frankenstein reinforced that.

"Lee W., congratulations on the appointment as chief. You've come a long way and I support you completely."

There was a brief uncomfortable pause on the phone, where after Lee W. thanked the man for his support.

"I wish I could say that this call was entirely about your appointment, Lee W. However, there is a transfer coming from the Wall's unit in Huntsville that I need to give you a head's up on."

"The Wall's unit? To the TDCJ?" Lee W. was familiar with the Wall's unit in Huntsville. Named for its red brick façade, it housed the death-row inmates and the execution chamber for the state of Texas. Here TDCJ stood for Texas Department of Criminal Justice, the prison hospital at the university.

"Yes. His name is Billie James Sampson. He's been on death row for rape and murder for about a year and a half. He has a solitary kidney and passes kidney stones. Right now, he is in acute renal failure from an obstructing stone in his ureter. Somehow they let him get so hyperkalemic that he had a grand-mal seizure" Here he referred to the elevated potassium and its relation to the seizure.

"Is he still seizing, Abbott?"

"No, he was treated by a decent fellow named Wilson, and seizure wise he is stable. But, unfortunately, he still has that stone and renal failure."

"Abbott, any reason for the solitary kidney?"

"Yes, there is the rub. Some general surgeon was taking care of him, doing open stone surgery and for some reason took out one of his kidneys. Some guy named Slim McCormick, any chance you know the guy? He practices out of Conroe Regional Medical Center."

"No, never heard of him. So, the patient has a solitary kidney that is obstructed by a ureteral stone in renal failure. I don't understand why you're involved, Abbott?"

"Well, turns out that this guy Wilson has some political clout and is raising holy hell. Claims that the removal of the kidney, which was the left one I think, was malpractice. You see the indication for its removal was just recurrent ureteral stones. I Guess Slim never thought about stone disease being generally bilateral." Frankenstein was here referring to the general finding that people that had recurrent stones usually passed these on both sides.

"Oh, oh. So, this is a delicate situation."

"Yes, it really is. Believe it or not, I got a phone call from the governor on this one just a few minutes ago. Seems that they really want us to use kid-gloves and try to not let the media get wind of this. Seems a real case of malpractice, but that can wait. So, Lee W., the internists are aware. I just got off the phone with Ben Adams, who will get the *fleas* on the case. But, I need urology to get involved quickly, yaw-all understand?" Here surprisingly

Frankenstein, a board-certified internist himself, referred to the slang used to address internists, namely flea in his reference to doctor Adams the head of internal medicine.

"Absolutely, Dana is here, in fact, I'll speak to her and get going on the case. He's probably going to need a perc-nephrostomy tube to cool down his renal function, and then we'll work up his stone disease and treat it appropriately."

"If you have any concerns don't hesitate to call me Lee W." As was the man's habit the phone went dead without a goodbye.

Lee W. returned to the great room and his guests. Everyone was interested in the phone call, so he decided to briefly explain about his new patient.

"That call was from Doctor Frankenstein."

There was a murmur in the room, the unique nature of the phone call appreciated by the largely medical group.

"We have a new patient, and he's quite a basket case. Billie James Sampson is visiting us from Huntsville courtesy of death row, the Walls unit. Seems as if he has a ureteral stone and a solitary kidney and is in renal failure. So, we're going to rent him a room and try to fix him up." There were some medically related questions which Lee W. answered, refraining from discussing the removal of his kidney. He then looked across the room at the chief resident.

Dana Rausch, MD was the urology service chief resident for the academic 1985-86 year. She was a very attractive woman of 33, with raven black hair typically worn in a tightly woven long ponytail trailing to her mid back. Then she was the hit of the party, especially with the wives, when she arrived, her hair stiffened with hairspray and backcombed into a big hair coiffure. She had a prominent widow's peak which gave her an interesting, intelligent look, with deep, dark, black eyes. She was a petite woman, dressed very conservatively in a navy-blue dress with matching heels.

"Dana, I need to talk to you. Could we adjourn to my study to discuss Mr. Sampson?"

Dana set her non-alcoholic drink down on a table and followed Lee W. In the study, he picked up a pile of medical journals to clear a space for her on a chair and sat behind his desk.

"What's up with this guy, Lee W.?" Dana said sitting.

"Ya, like I said a real basket case."

"Ya…I get the idea; Frankenstein calls you at home. At what?" She looked at her watch. "It's midnight, what's the deal?"

"Like I said he has a stone in the ureter and a solitary kidney. Now there is the problem, and we need to keep this as quiet as possible. If any media contact you, refer them to me. Anyway, some idiot in Sam Houston took out his other kidney."

"So, the remaining kidney now is obstructed, and you said he is in renal failure?"

"Ya, with hyperkalemia and a grand-mal seizure. Now, take a look at him. Probably going to need a perc to cool him down." Here he referred to a percutaneous nephrostomy tube that would be inserted by radiology through the skin and into the kidney. This procedure would relieve the pressure on the kidney and let the renal failure resolve. "Get the intern to see him first, but I think we need to get going on this tonight. Get this! The governor just called Frankenstein about this case."

"The governor? Didn't think democrats stayed up this late!"

"Ya, there are real problems with this surgeon who is a general surgeon named Slim McCormack. They don't want the media to get wind of this, the guy is in real legal trouble."

"Why's this guy on death row?"

"Only murder and rape. The guy is a real piece of work. Now yaw-all be careful with this guy."

Chapter 3

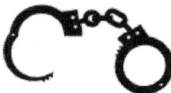

Dana left the party a few minutes later with a take-home box of Jill's Diner's famous apple pie for the intern who was to meet her in the urology library. The wind blew, a storm approaching in the Gulf reported on the static-filled radio as she drove her red, rusted, 1968 VW bug. When she got out of the car, she forgot the pie.

"We need to get his films, Mark. I had some pie for you from the party but of course, left it in my car. I'll get it for you later today."

Mark Upham MD was the urology service intern. He was a tall, balding man with brown hair, a big friendly smile, and small round wire-rim glasses. He pointed to a large x-ray jacket on the floor below the x-ray view box. "Got them from Huntsville for you, chief."

"Great!" Dana walked to the front of the library. She sat first, took her heels off and replaced them with some white Rebook shoes with pink laces. "Ahhhh," she sighed in response to the shoe change. Then she was back up, grabbing the x-ray jacket. "When was his nephrectomy?" Here she wondered when the left kidney had been removed.

"Last month," Mark said with a little chuckle. "And now he's in renal failure."

"Is he still? Do we have his labs?"

Mark read from a paper filled white plastic clipboard. His creatinine is elevated at 4, it was 3.2 yesterday." Here he referred to the serum creatinine which inversely measures kidney function with normal being less than 1 mg per deciliter. These numbers were high and getting higher over time. "His potassium was 5.9 his uric acid was, get this 15, before his seizure, with the glucose and insulin the potassium is down to 4.1."

"Okay, let's look at his rays." She went through the x-ray jacket and pulled out an intravenous pyelogram (IVP) from September 1985. This is a study where dye is given intravenously, the kidney picks up the dye and excretes it giving a picture of the inside of the kidney. "Now here he has two kidneys, so it's before the nephrectomy. Look at this," she said pointing to the left kidney image. "The KUB shows what I think is medullary sponge kidney (MSK). It is most obvious by far in the left kidney. See the *paintbrush* appearance of calcifications over the medulla of the kidney? That's MSK. Now look, there is much less but some of that change is seen over the right kidney. Did he not pass right sided stones?"

"He says…with very little conversation I should say, that he passed left sided stones repeatedly his entire adult life, but on a rare occasion had a right-sided episode."

"With this x-ray and his history, I would have never taken out the left kidney unless it was non-functional and this IVP shows that it excretes dye." If a kidney excretes dye it is relatively healthy, certainly not non-functional.

"Here is a KUB from today, Dana."

Dana put the film up on the view box. She took out a plastic ruler and measured the stone. As she talked she brushed her hair back and was able to get it into a semblance of a ponytail secured with a hair tie. "There is a seven to eight-millimeter stone overlying the right mid ureter. There are definite MSK changes in the right kidney. Now we need to have the radiologist put a perc-nephrostomy tube in ASAP. They will want anesthesia to monitor him during the procedure. So, set that up. Tonight, if possible. That will treat his renal failure and then we can deal with the stone. "Let's go meet the ... let's just say challenged patient."

"I don't know Dana. He is a very tough, very unfriendly guy. Be careful around him!"

The TDCJ hospital, just nicknamed the TDCJ, was built in July 1983. It was a nine-floor hospital to 172 inpatient beds, a multi-service ambulatory care center, a minor operating room with a recovery room, a telemetry 12-bed unit, a medical intensive care unit of 6 beds and a 56-bed overnight holding unit. It was staffed by Texas Department of Criminal Justice Institutional Division officers.

The TDCJ was attached to John Sealy hospital by an overhead wire covered walkway on the third floor that gives little protection from the hard rain of the developing storm when the two made their way across the walkway and checked into the prison hospital. Once in the TDCJ, they were faced with a different world of gray painted walls and correctional officers.

Officer Thomas sat at a wire screened check-in cage looking threatening in his gray and black uniform. "Can I help you?" There was an atmosphere of indifferent oblivion that was evident from the moment that you exited the walkway and entered TDCJ characterized by this officer. "I am Doctor Rausch and this is Doctor Upham, we are here to see the inpatient Billie James Sampson."

"Sorry, the facility is closed at this time. Please return during operating hours of 8 AM to 7 PM," the officer said in a rote manner. He forced a smile on his face as two uniformed officers arrived to escort the physicians out of the facility.

"Wait, we have orders from Doctor Abbott Frankenstein, the university president. We need to see this patient." With some force, the two officers grabbed their elbows and deposited them outside in the walkway.

Rain beat down on them as they realized that no access was the standard of the day. "Come on," Dana said as the two ran down the walkway to dry ground in the John Sealy hospital, looking for a phone.

"Lee W., so sorry to bother you at home but they say the TDCJ is closed until 8 AM. I wanted to see the man and arrange for that perc."

"Gosh, that unit is impossible. Wait till you see the patients and find they are nicer than the guards. I'll call Bill Ramport the director of TDCJ and get back to you."

"Let's go back to the library, pick up the x-ray jacket, and go over to radiology and arrange that perc," Dana said.

As they were talking to the interventional radiology resident on call, a page from Lee W. came to Dana's beeper. Picking up a phone she said: "Lee W., what happened?"

"Go back over and talk to officer Thomas. Ramport spoke to him, and he will let you in."

"Thomas is the one I talked to and wouldn't let me in, Lee W."

"He will now."

"Officer Thomas, I believe Doctor Ramport has approved our entry."

The man looked down at his paperwork. "Your names?"

"I'm Dana Rausch this is Mark Upham."

The officer studied his paperwork for the longest time. Eventually, he made a quiet phone call and unintelligibly spoke to the person on the other end of the call. He looked up and said: "Just a moment." The same two officers arrived and escorted them through security. Each looked closely at Dana's shoes. Here they were then "buzzed" through the main door, the sound menacing and final. The officers led them to the elevator and to the fourth-floor nursing station. After reading the patient's chart, they moved to his room. He had been put in isolation involving a single room, two officers at the doors with guns and cuff-link tie-clasps.

"Mr. Sampson, I am Doctor Dana Rausch, the urology chief resident, this is Doctor Mark Upham, our intern." Dana stuck out her hand to shake.

Mr. Sampson sat on his bed staring at her with his steel blue eyes without emotion and did not meet her grip. "You don't look like an Indian chief." He said a small smile quietly revealing golden dentation. "Maybe a little Indian in your blood, where's yaw-all war paint?"

Dana overlooked the patient's comment. Sampson kept his blue eyes on the girl to an uncomfortable point. There was a sexual tension exuded by the man in his dealing with Dana, he just ignored Mark Upham. She decided in her mind to limit the questions to those important ones.

"Have you ever had a right-sided stone, Mr. Sampson?"

Sampson just shrugged his shoulder. "Maybe one or two."

"Can I see your incisions?" There was a long quiet spell while Sampson just stared at the woman. She reluctantly moved to the patient's left side and pulled up his gown to reveal a healed left flank incision, several healed incisions in the left abdomen, and a huge eagle chest tattoo. When she went to palpate the incision Sampson put a hand gently on her wrist. She pulled her hand away. "Please don't touch me!"

Sampson smiled that small smile and said nothing staring at the woman.

Dana moved to the patient's right side, no incisions were seen. She lightly tapped the right flank with her fist, the patient silently grimacing. A similar tap on his left side was painless.

"Mr. Sampson."

"Billie," he said slowly with his small smile and gold teeth visible.

"I prefer Mr. Sampson," she said. "Radiology is going to put a tube in through your skin about right here," pointing to the right flank. "The tube is called a percutaneous nephrostomy and will relieve the obstruction in your right kidney. They should be doing this soon. When was your last meal?"

Sampson just shrugged his shoulders.

The procedure was monitored by anesthesia. A page during it revealed that the patient would not sign a legal consent to allow the procedure and that he insisted on having Dana do the procedure.

"Mr. Sampson, you need to sign the consent allowing us to do this procedure. It is important to get you out of kidney failure."

"Last time I's sign I's lost a kidney, Dana." This was the first time that the patient had used her first name, its use very uncomfortable. "I'm Doctor Rausch, Mr. Sampson!"

"Why did I's lose a kidney, Doctor?"

"Just sign will you and forget me doing the procedure. I have no experience doing these."

Sampson said: "Did Slim have experience?"

Chapter 4

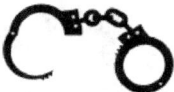

The percutaneous nephrostomy tube was placed in Billie James Sampson by the interventional radiologist in the middle of the night. Anesthesia stood by in case of a recurrent seizure, but the procedure went flawlessly, the patient did well. This tube was inserted through the skin and into the kidney allowing the obstructed urine to drain, correcting the cause of his renal failure. He was safe and sound in the TDCJ, waiting for the group.

Rounds began, as usual, the next morning at 6:30 AM on the urology ward, west three B (W3B). The crowd included the chief resident Dana Rauch, her hair now devoid of hairspray and woven, as usual, into a tight ponytail. She was dressed in green scrubs with a white jacket thrown over and her rebook OR shoes.

The group included senior resident Duke McHugh, intern Mark Upham, and the two new medical students, all dressed in ties and dresses with sweeping white coats, pockets jammed with stethoscopes, percussion hammers, and paper notes.

Miss Bonnie was the W3B ward clerk, a UTMB employee for over 40 years. She was an African-American woman, stick thin with straightened black hair pulled back in a bun. She had mile-long curved, exotically painted fingernails, this week all ten battle flags of the Confederacy. She took care of the urologists but was someone you should not cross. Today she gathered the service's charts and placed them in a wire-wheeled basket labeled *Stream Team*. Pushing the basket, the entourage gathered in front of the first patient's room.

The group surrounded the intern waiting for the presentations to begin. "Mr. Marcum is now seven days' status-post radical cystectomy and ileal loop." Here Upham described a man one week after an operation where the bladder and lymph nodes were removed for bladder cancer, each kidney's ureter connected to a loop of bowel brought to the skin as a stoma called an ileal loop. "He's been afebrile, his vital signs stable. His lungs are clear and, here's the punch-line, he had flatus!"

The group was excited, showing this with mock cheers. Patient's after major abdominal surgery like a radical cystectomy, do not get intestinal movement for some time after surgery, a condition called an ileus. Things such as flatus, the passage of gas, mark resolution of that condition and in this patient celebrated because it had been a whole week.

"Does he have good bowel sounds?" Dana asked the typical follow-up question of the intern.

"He's got some tinkles," was the man's response.

"Let's go see him."

Within the room was a middle-aged Caucasian male sleeping in a hospital bed. When the group entered, he woke, elevating the head of his bed, turning on the bedside light, and putting in his hearing aids. "Hi, doctor Rausch," the man said sleepily. "Did you hear the good news?" Everyone in the group clapped quietly.

"Yes, congratulations Mr. Marcum. Shall we try you on some liquids?"

"I can't wait; can I get a breakfast?"

"Just liquids at first. Are you up and walking."

"Three times in the hall yesterday."

Dana moved to the bedside, pulled up the covers, and pulled back the man's gown. His incision was judged to be healing well, the stoma healthy.

In the hallway, Dana began dictating directions to the group. "Okay, Mark start him on clear liquids. Get the stoma nurse to take one stent out today and the other tomorrow with a shot of gentamycin with each." Here she referred to the removal of a long tube called a stent which was up in the kidney, the ends visible in the stoma. After each removal, the patient would receive an injection of an antibiotic to prevent seeding the bloodstream with bacteria.

As they talked, Lee W. came hustling down the hall joining the group. He was dressed in a pink button-down collared shirt with a brown and blue tie, and khaki pants worn over an orange pair of iguana skin cowboy boots. "Hi yaw-all, Dana, how's Mr. Marcum? He's one week today, right?"

"Ya, he's got flatus and were starting him on clear liquids, taking out a stent today."

"Mind if I round with you? Afterward, I want to go over to the TDCJ with just you Dana," Lee W. said to the woman quietly.

The group made their way seeing each of the twenty or so patients on the urology service, leaving the TDCJ till last. "Let's go to radiology and see Mr. Sampson's nephrostogram."

Doctor Chad Finkelstein was the interventional radiologist that placed the tube in Mr. Sampson's kidney during the night. He was a tall thin man with a bowl of curly brown hair, a slight separation of his two front teeth, and thick round horn-rimmed glasses. He sat in a darkened room at a large mechanized view box with multiple x-rays when the group arrived.

"Chad, you got the films from last night?"

Finkelstein looked at the group, now standing around him. "You mean on Sampson?"

"Ya, the nephrostogram," Dana said.

"That guy's a piece of work, Dana. Meanest guy I think I've ever worked on. Thought he was going to bite me. I didn't use much lidocaine I'll say."

"One of Texas' finest," Dana responded.

"Yaw-all I won't tell you what he said about you!"

"Yes, please don't."

Finkelstein placed several nephrostogram x-rays on the view box. As he did he glanced at Dana and smiled. The films showed the procedure where the tube was placed into the kidney and dye injected into the collecting system.

"The system was quite hydronephrotic when we entered it." Here he referred to the dilation of the collecting system reflecting obstruction of urine flow. "Here's the initial nephrostogram. Here's the stone in the mid-ureter about seven millimeters in diameter." With a telescopic pointer, he pointed out a density overlying the mid-ureter of the kidney.

"Yaw-all, this is Mr. Sampson. He's a guy in renal failure with an obstructed right kidney." Lee W. went on to question the medical students. "Lee, why would a guy be in renal failure with only one obstructed kidney?"

Lee Mathis was a young black male medical student with a short Afro haircut and black glasses. "Well, the only reason would be that the other kidney is non-functioning."

"Or absent, you're right, one obstructed kidney does not explain renal failure." He pointed to the area of the right kidney. Here were calcifications, *paintbrush*-like overlying the medulla or middle of the kidney. "Linda, what is the cause of his stone disease.?"

Linda Fellows was a young medical student with curly blonde hair and excited shiny blue eyes. "Well, you're describing these as *paintbrush* like, I think that refers to medullary sponge kidney, right?"

"Ya, that's the diagnosis. Duke, tell the group about the disease."

Duke McHugh, MD was a tall, heavy-set Caucasian man, senior resident in his fourth year of post-graduate training. He was aware more than most of Lee W.'s tendency to pimp or question the students and residents on rounds, or any other time in fact. Luckily, he knew a great deal about the relatively common disorder. "Well, medullary sponge kidney, also known as Cacchi–Ricci disease, is a relatively common cause of recurrent stone disease. It is congenital, that is the patient was born with it and tends to run in families. It is generally bilateral, that is in both kidneys. The disorder is based upon cystic dilations in the tubules of the kidney where urine collects and calcium precipitates out as a stone. These stones then drop out of the collecting system to give recurrent renal colic episodes."

"Okay, well what do you think we do with this stone, Dana?" Lee W. pointed at the stone with his index finger.

"It's in the mid-ureter, quite high for ureteroscopic extraction, but worth a try."
Here the chief resident was referring to a procedure where a telescope is placed into the bladder and then retrograde, up the ureter to the stone. In 1985 this procedure was new, and the presence of the stone quite high in the mid-ureter made it quite unlikely to be successful. "I'd give it a try though, with a ureteralithotomy if we aren't successful." Here she described a plan of giving the ureteroscope a trial but if not successful, then an open removal of the stone with an incision would be performed. "We need to let his renal failure cool down, however." The renal failure which was secondary to obstruction of the kidney was now been treated with the percutaneous nephrostomy tube, and the plan would be to leave the tube until completely treated.

"Correct, we need to let the drainage of the kidney occur and have him stabilize. He had a seizure because of hyperkalemia."

Here Lee W. reminded the group of the patient's seizure from elevated potassium. Lee W. turned to Mark Upham the intern. "Mark, what was his creatinine and potassium this morning, do you know?"

"Yes," he turned and flipped through his clipboard. "Mr. Sampson's morning creatinine was back to normal at 1.2 mg per deciliter, his potassium was normal." Here the intern referred to the serum creatinine, a measure of kidney function, the lower the better normal being about 1.2 with one kidney.

"Okay, well thanks for the films and the job last night, Chad."

As was his tendency, he responded to the group: "Now you're talking Hebrew."

The group broke up. Duke went to the OR. He had several cystoscopic cases to do, that is cases involving placing a scope in the bladder of the patient. Mark Upham had a whole slew of scut work to do from rounds. The medical students had classes and clinics to man. Dana and Lee W. went to the TDCJ.

It was still stormy outside, rain and wind quite prominent on the walkway to the TDCJ. The two ran shielding themselves from the torrent with their hands. They were buzzed into the facility and stood shaking off the rain at the front desk and officer Thomas.

"We're here to see Mr. Sampson."

"ID's please," officer Thomas asked of the two physicians. He stared for a moment at Dana's rebook shoes.

Both showed their UTMB picture cards and were led into the facility. The TDCJ has 172 individual patient beds, some semi-private, many as with Mr. Sampson private rooms. At the door were two armed guards, dressed in gray and black, each with handcuff tie clasps and black sunglasses. Lee W. nodded to the men as the two walked into the room.

Inside the room was Mr. Sampson dressed in only pajama bottoms, his eagle tattooed chest visible for all. There was a dressing on his right flank with a tube going to a bag hung from the bedside.

"Mr. Sampson, how are you this morning?" Dana said to the prisoner. She kept some distance between herself and the patient.

Sampson said nothing. He looked at Lee W. wondering who he was.

"Mr. Sampson, I am doctor Hickok, the chief of urology. Are you doing okay this morning?"

Sampson said nothing at first but shook his head affirmatively. "You look more like an Indian chief. She looks like a squaw. When do I get breakfast?" He said quietly.

Lee W. stepped forward. "Okay, let's stop all this Indian squaw business. Yaw-all, Dr. Rausch is your physician. She should be called Dr. Rausch, and nothing else. Do you understand?"

Sampson sat in his bed quietly staring at the two. "Okay, Dr. Rausch and Dr. Hickok, when do I eat? And by the way, when would I pee?"

Lee W. looked at Dana. "Well he's not in renal failure anymore, a regular diet perhaps sodium restricted would be in order. What type of urine output did he put out through that nephrostomy tube?"

Lee W. grabbed the bedside chart. "5 liters since last night, quite a post-obstructive diuresis." Here he referred to the output in urine from the nephrostomy tube since its placement. An obstructive kidney when that obstruction is relieved will often put out an inappropriate amount of urine over the next day.

"Your urine output is coming out through the tube, Mr. Sampson." Dana picked up the urine bag from the bed rail. "You probably won't void much until we get rid of the stone."

"When do I get rid of the stone?" There was still a quiet antagonism between the patient and doctors. "When do I get my left kidney back?" The man looked first at Lee W. and then at Dana with those steel blue dead set eyes. "Yaw-all can do things like that, can't you?"

Chapter 5

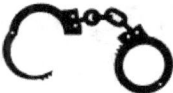

Sampson's last remark set a pallor over the two. Something was brewing in the patient's mind. It was thought that even Sampson did not think re-implantation of the kidney was possible. He had a twisted scowl of vengeance on his gold-toothed face when he mentioned it. To settle the subject, the kidney was long ago dead, soaked in formalin and sliced up by the pathologist in Conroe. Renal transplants are for people with chronic renal failure, not with a functioning renal unit. In addition, his life expectancy, remember lethal injection awaited him in the near future, was not a great characteristic to have when thinking about renal transplant surgery.

Lee W. left Dana and moved on to his office. He was anxious to get to his new workplace and begin straightening things out. His old office was small, now the chairmanship and the chairman's office were all his. What awaited him put a hold on his desires?

"They wouldn't wait in the waiting room, Lee W.!" Lee W. inherited Sarah Jones as his personal secretary during the transition. She was a very efficient, pleasant, woman, somewhat overweight but pretty in a Texas manner. "I tried to make them comfortable in the waiting room, but their lawyers and they you know insisted Lee W." She was frightened of what her new boss would say, not really knowing the man yet.

"There's two lawyers in my office, Sarah?"

"Yes, boss. So sorry, I tried."

Lee W. entered his new office. It was a large square shaped room with a large cherry wood desk, a large picture window looking out at 'ole Red" the original medical school building, and a sitting area with couch. The two lawyers were sitting on his sofa sipping coffee from porcelain cups. They both stood up upon his entrance and introduced themselves.

"I am Luther Jackson," a tall black man with cornrow hairstyle said as he shook Lee W.'s hand.

"I'm Felix Artain," a shorter white man with balding head and thick black glasses.

"Let's sit down here and talk. Do yaw-all have enough coffee?"

Both indicated that they were okay. "We, my partner and I, am representing William James Sampson. He claims that his left kidney was removed from him in an inappropriate manner. What is your opinion on this.?"

Lee W. thought hard about his answer. MSK is generally a bilateral condition but can be unilateral. The history as he understood it, was that the patient always passed stones from the left kidney. Evidently, there was some distant history of stones passage on the right.

"I don't know. Medullary sponge kidney is the diagnosis for the reason he has stones. While that is usually bilateral it can be unilateral   I think Dr. McCormack assumed it to be only unilateral."

"Well, it's obviously a bilateral condition, now with the obstruction of his right kidney and renal failure with a seizure." Felix Artain stood as if addressing a judge, as he made his case.

Lee W. thought about the men. He wondered about their backgrounds, probably like most malpractice lawyers some knowledge of medicine, but mostly just of the law. "Well let's wait. Perhaps he will drop no further stones down that right ureter."

"What is the plan for our client?"

"Well, yaw-all know that this is medicine and we take one step at a time. First thing is to get his renal failure to cool down with the nephrostomy tube. Then in a few days, we will go to the OR and try to remove the stone through the bladder with what's called a ureteroscope. If that is not successful then in the same sitting do an open stone surgery and remove the stone, a ureteralithotomy that your client is familiar with."

There was something in the air, some problem that the two lawyers were having difficulty voicing. Lee W. could sense it but hoped to get the two out of his office. "Yaw-all I've got a million things to do. If you all would please excuse me," he said gathering the two together and directing them to the door.

"We have another subject that we must discuss Dr. Hickok." Luther Jackson turned and made his way back to the couch. He said over his shoulder: "My client wants you to personally take care of him. He is not happy about what is her name, Dana Rausch." The two lawyers sat on the couch. Both picked up cups and finished their coffee.

Anger flashed in Lee W. He grabbed a chair and plunked it down and sat in front of the two lawyers. "Wait a minute, this is a teaching institution and we do not have private patient's here. Dr. Rausch is a capable member of our team, chief resident for heavens' sake. She will be taking care of this patient. Is this understood? Make it clear to your client that she is the number one member of his team without exception!"

The two put their cups down on the coffee table. "I'll try to emphasize that to Mr. Sampson." Mr. Artain said with some hesitation in his voice.

Lee W. was now nearly yelling. "Also." He calmed himself and continued to speak firmly. "This idea that the left kidney could somehow be re-transplanted is bogus. Make sure he realizes that that option is out."

"Why is that?" Mr. Jackson spoke up.

Let me tell you a million reasons. First, your client is a dirt-bag and on death row, Lee W. thought. "Are you," Lee W. wanted to use the word crazy. Instead, he chose the word *unwise*. "Are

51

you...unwise," he said now totally in control. "Mr. Sampson's left kidney was removed weeks ago. It was dead at the time of removal, fixed in formalin, and cut up by the pathologist. It's gone, no hero rescues here."

"But certainly, he is a candidate for a cadaveric or living related donor transplant. Mr. Sampson has a loving brother in Dallas."

"Ya, I bet he does. A renal transplant is for, and only for, those people with chronic renal failure not with one good kidney. You need to read up on the subject." Lee W. stood and motioned the two off of the couch. "Now with that, yaw-all I must insist I have a clinic to see patients."

Lee W. ushered them to the door. He shook their hands and said: "now remember, no further nonsense about doctor Rausch."

The day was for arranging his office, but it did not turn out that way. He was beginning to realize the job of chief was not just a clinical one.

"Doctor Hickok, a Jennifer Harry is at the desk wanting to talk to you. She says her Dad is your patient and *oh-by-the-way* she continues on about being a reporter with KTRK that you have interacted with before."

"What does she want to talk about, do you know?"

"Mr. Sampson!"

"Okay, give me a couple of minutes then invite her in Sarah." Lee W. took that time to straighten up his office, pushing cardboard boxes to the side of the room, straightening up his desk, and one last thing. He sat at his desk and retrieved the hidden key from behind his credenza, opening the lower desk drawer. Before him was his last empty bottle of Jim Beam Bourbon, Sweet Amber. In days past this would have been full and in his mouth about now, but he was 47 and ½ months sober and its presence gave him peace somehow. He took the bottle in his hand, opened the cap, and took a deep breath through his nose. There wasn't much of a smell left, but it calmed his nerves.

There was a knock on the door. Lee W. replaced the bottle and closed the drawer with the toe of his boot. "Yes, come in."

"Hello, doctor Hickok." In stepped a tall black girl with a short afro dressed in a pink pullover sweatshirt with a white-edged hood, freshly iron denim jeans, and brown deck shoes. She pulled a leopard skin backpack off of her back and set it down by the wall. In her hand was a small notebook and pencil. "I hope you remember me, I am Jennifer Harry, you're my father's urologist. You saved his life. Can I give you a hug?"

After a quick embrace, Lee W. asked? "Yes, how is Dupree doing? I haven't seen him in a while I think." Dupree Harry was an elderly man with metastatic prostate cancer doing well after undergoing an orchiectomy or removal of the testicles. Prior to the procedure, the man was near death with widespread prostate cancer metastasis and an unusual case of clotting abnormalities seen rarely in prostate cancer called DIC or disseminated intravascular coagulation. The minor procedure of testicle removal put all of his disease in remission and resolved his bleeding problem.

"He's doing amazing. I think he sees you next week. He really is doing well after that surgery that you did on him. Like magic really."

"Good. What can I do for you today?" Lee W. had an omen, he knew that he was going to get hammered about Mr. Sampson.

"Well, here is my card," she said pulling a card from her back pocket and setting it on Lee W.'s desk. "I didn't know if you remembered my association with KTRK and the Galveston County Daily News?"

"Oh ya, I remember well. J.T. Splintter and that fiasco associated with his death, and then didn't you cover the Maloney death?" Lee W. referred to the death of the governor of Texas J.T.Splintter after surgery and the death of the heiress Siobhan Maloney at a fraternity party.

"Guilty of both." There was a long pause in the room. "Well, doctor Hickok I wanted to ask you some questions about Billie James Sampson a guy from TDCJ and the Wall's unit who was admitted to UTMB with kidney stones."

"I am very familiar with that patient Jennifer, but you know patient confidentiality keeps me from saying much."

"Can you confirm that you are treating him for kidney stones?"

Lee W. thought about the question. It was general information that he had been treated for recurrent stones. "Yes, but that is all I can confirm right now."

"Can you confirm that he has only one kidney and that the other kidney was removed by doctor McCormick of Sam Houston Texas?"

"Woo…I can't discuss his case any further Jennifer!"

"Was he in kidney failure?"

"Can't say, Jennifer."

"Okay, I understand." She said as she picked up her backpack stuffing her notebook in the side pocket.

They made small talk mostly about her Dad's case and then she left. "Thank you for your time, doctor Hickok."

Lee W. sat at his desk for a moment. He picked up the phone and spoke to Sarah. "Sarah, get Abbott Frankenstein on the phone for me sometime this morning."

Chapter 6

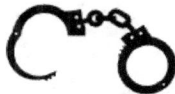

The phone call did not go through until early afternoon.

"Lee W., how is Sampson doing." Doctor Frankenstein had a big booming voice which matched his body habitus and name, tall at six foot seven.

"Well, he is doing fine, Abbott. His perc nephrostomy tube was successfully placed by interventional radiology and his creatinine is down to 1.2, his potassium and uric acid have normalized. I had a visit from KTRK this morning, however. They seem to be on the case and the basic details. I said really nothing based on patient privacy."

"Good, try not to speak to them. Who was the reporter, Jennifer Harry?"

"Yes, I take care of her father and it seems as if it gains her access to me whenever."

"Well, she is a good reporter, and UTMB seems to be on her beat. She is always around when less than attractive medical things happen. I know you know her, but do not give out Sampson information. You did a good job. Talk to Lloyd Thomas the shift sergeant. He for all intense and purposes runs the TDCJ." And like that he practiced his usual behavior and hung up the phone devoid of a salutation.

Lee W. looked at the end of his receiver, the dial-tone now blaring. "Sarah, call the TDCJ and find out the latest that I can talk to an Officer Lloyd Thomas today. I need to walk over and see him, but want to do some work in my office first."

"Yes, Doctor Hickok."

Lee W. walked over to the TDCJ at 4:30 pm that afternoon. The storm was still present but rain was not falling as he made his way along the walkway to the prison. He walked into the building and stood at the front desk.

Sitting at the desk was a large white man dressed in the gray and black TDCJ uniform with a brass name badge that said, Officer Huckster. "I'm Doctor Hickok, Doctor Frankenstein asked me to speak to the shift sergeant, Officer Thomas." The man looked up from his paperwork and looked at Lee W. He said just one word: "I/D."

Lee W. reached to his white coat and removed the picture I/D badge and handed it to Officer Huckster. The man said nothing scanning the card as if he was looking for fingerprints. He then tossed the badge back at Lee W., and pointed to his right, a room with drawn blinds and a big black door.

Within the room was an overweight woman with a nineteen-fiftyish curled and waved cut blonde hair, red mid-calf cut suit, chewing gum. Lee W. stopped in front of her desk, read her name tag and addressed her as Robyn. "Robyn, I'm Doctor Hickok, Doctor Frankenstein asked me to speak to shift sergeant, Officer Thomas."

"It's Rob…yen."

"What?"

"It's Rob…yen, the y, pronounce the y."

"Oh…Rob…yen?"

"Yes. I/D."

Lee W. thought about Officer Huckster's exam of his badge, but took it off his white coat and handed it to the woman. As with the officer, she examined the badge carefully. The woman returned the badge and pointed to a big black door to her left. "Please knock."

Lee W. knocked quietly on the door. A voice said: "come in."

Within the room was a gray metal desk piled high with files. Officer Thomas was barely visible sitting behind the clutter. He was a black man in his fifties, with a short buzzed haircut, dressed in gray and black. He looked up with a scowl and said nothing.

"Officer Thomas, I'm Doctor Hickok, Doctor Frankenstein asked me to speak to you."

"I/D," was the one-word answer. Lee W. had not put the badge back on his coat thinking that he would be quizzed again and handed it to the man. Again, close examination of the badge was noted. Thomas handed the badge back to Lee W. and said nothing staring at him.

"Officer Thomas, Doctor Frankenstein asked me to speak to you."

"You said that!"

"Well, the subject is an inmate in the TDCJ, Mr. Billie James Sampson."

"What about him?" He said moving files around the desk and not looking at Lee W.

Lee W. sighed to himself. "Well, Doctor Frankenstein and I want to touch bases with you about the patient."

Again without looking up he said: "you mean inmate?"

"Yes, the inmate Sampson. As you know he has some urologic problems and we are treating him."

"What's the point?"

"Well, I was contacted by the media. A Jennifer Harry of KTRK and the Galveston Daily, and she had a lot of information about the patient that we would rather not be out in the media."

For the first time, the officer looked up at Lee W. "And you think that leak came from the TDCJ?"

"Well, no I didn't mean that."

"What did you mean?"

"I wanted to touch bases about the issue. For medical reasons we want any media attention about this patient funneled through the president's office, or…through me….it could go through me."

"You mean inmate."

"Yes, inmate."

Thomas stood, and pulled up his pants over his substantial paunch. "Mr. Hickok, I am very busy as you can see. I can assure you that the information that Miss Harry has did not come and won't come from here." He walked around the desk and put a hand on Lee W. directing him to the door. "Now if you will excuse me."

The next morning Lee W. did what he always does. In his boxer shorts and wife beater shirt, he stood on his front porch and retrieved the Galveston Daily. Below the fold on the front page were headlines that shocked him.

The article, titled: Death Row Inmate Treated at UTMB. The article went on to state that the inmate was in kidney failure from kidney stones. The presence of those stones were confirmed by Doctor Lee W. Hickok. It went on to discuss the removal of his opposite kidney by Doctor James "Slim" McCormack of Conroe

Texas. Other than the reference to kidney stones, Lee W. was not quoted. The rest of the article relied on "anonymous sources."

Lee W. turned around and went into his house. He blasted upstairs to his office. Rummaging around he finally found Jennifer Harry's card. He dialed her office phone number, getting an answering machine. "Hello, this is Jennifer Harry. At the tone leave a message."

"Jennifer this is Doctor Hickok. I just read your Galveston Daily article. Call me ASAP at, and he dictated his phone number."

Lee W. sat at his desk staring. He was so upset, who did she get to confirm those facts? He wondered if Frankenstein would hold him responsible. Could a student or resident have talked to her? He had a feeling that the leak was in the TDCJ, but he couldn't be certain. The phone rang.

"Hello."

"Doctor Hickok, it's Jennifer Harry. I got your message. What's up?"

"That article, where did you get that information."

"I can't tell you my sources, but they are reliable. Was anything in that article not true?"

Lee W. thought before answering. "No, but I'm the only named source. Looks like you got the information from me."

"I sourced anonymous sources except for your confirmation of kidney stones."

"Yes, but…we really hoped that the information, especially about McCormack, would not be reported."

"Why's that?"

"I can't really say."

"Well, we're at an impasse then. I can't tell you my source. They are reliable, however."

Lee W. paged Dana. "Dana, Lee W. We have a problem. Have you seen this morning's Galveston Daily?"

"No. No time Lee W. What's up?"

"A reporter named Jennifer Harry wrote an article on our friend, Mr. Sampson. She is the daughter of a patient of mine. The article indicates that he is in renal failure and that the kidney was removed by Slim. Any idea who leaked the info?"

There was silence on the other end. "Is she a young black girl?"

"Yes, that's her did you speak to her?"

"She tried to interview me and Duke in the cafeteria. We both said nothing and referred her to you like you told us."

"Well, Slim McCormack may be in trouble."

"Is that our problem, really?"

"Well, Frankenstein wanted this to remain in the university, but I don't know, we haven't done anything wrong so maybe not. I'll be in my office in ten minutes, meet me there, I want to go see Sampson."

When he hung up the phone rang immediately. "Hello."

"Lee W., Abbott Frankenstein. Did you see the paper?"

Chapter 7

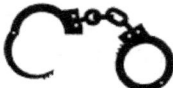

It was cystoscopy morning clinic for Lee W. Dressed in scrubs and brown ostrich skinned boots, he performed examinations on ten patients, one after the other. The procedure involved placing a telescope retrograde into the bladder through the urethra. Here the inside of the urethra, prostate, and bladder could then be examined under local anesthesia.

He finished his last patient and entered his office. Sitting on the couch as planned was Dana Rausch. He paged her to meet him here at 10 AM.

For the first time in days she was not dressed in scrubs for the OR, but rather wore a sleeveless white modestly scooped collar blouse worn over a knee-length red skirt with low heeled black shoes. Her white coat sat by her side. Her hair was pulled back into her usual tight weaved ponytail.

"Hi, Dana. Let me just write a quick note on this patient before I forget." Lee W. sat at his desk, now crowded with patient charts, and wrote a note about the findings of the last cystoscopy. As he penned, he spoke to the woman. "I want to round with you at the TDCJ and see Sampson."

The word rounds refer to a physician or physicians seeing patients on the service. For the urology service, Dana conducted formal rounds in the morning before surgery at 6:30 Am. She would follow this with afternoon rounds after surgery, around 4:30 PM. These were working rounds where, as the chief resident, she would make decisions on patient care and discharge. Attending those rounds would be the resident, intern, and medical students.

Lee W. generally left those rounds to the residents but was making it a habit of seeing Mr. Sampson at least once a day with Dana. If the truth was known, he was somewhat afraid of the man, not to himself, but rather for his chief resident, a petite and very beautiful woman. Mr. Sampson, a cold-blooded killer.

"Have you seen Sampson's morning KUB, Dana?" Here he referred to a plain x-ray of the abdomen.

"Yes, the stone is still in the mid-right ureter, the tube is an adequate position. His creatinine this morning is down to 0.8." He was now three days after placement of the right nephrostomy tube. The tube had done what it was designed to do, decompress the pressure in the kidney and bring his kidney function back to normal as measured by the normal creatinine level.

Lee W. stood and stretched. He gathered the charts and put them in his outbox. He moved to the coat rack near his door and retrieved his white coat. The two then went walking away.

"Let's stop in x-ray and let me get a look at that KUB." Lee W. asked of his chief resident.

The front desk of the x-ray department quickly found Sampson's KUB and gave it to the two physicians. Lee W. threw the film upon a view box.

He pointed to the stone, unmoved still in the mid ureter, with his telescopic pen. A small tube was visible entering the flank and curling in the area of the kidney's renal pelvis, the funnel portion of the kidney and represented the nephrostomy tube. Multiple *paintbrush* like calcifications were seen overlying the kidney from the patient's active stone disease.

"I think he is ready for surgery; Lee W. Should I put him on the schedule for tomorrow?"

"That is what I was thinking. Today, while I'm there, I want you to get a consent from him. It would be for ureteroscopic stone extraction and possible open ureteralithotomy." Here the plan would be to go through the urethra to the bladder with a small scope called a ureteroscope and try to pull the stone down and out the bladder. Failing that they would make an incision and remove the stone, a procedure called ureteralithotomy. "Be real complete with the man, and then write or dictate a detailed note about the patient's consent." A consent documents that the surgeon tells the patient about the surgery and possible risks and benefits.

The two walked over to the TDCJ. There was beautiful sunny daylight in the walkway, quite a contrast from the days before. They entered the facility, stopping at the front desk.

Officer Camden looked up from his desk and eyed them suspiciously. He checked first Lee W. and then Dana from head to foot, stopping to examine Dana's shoes particularly. Both Lee W.

and Dana pulled their I/D badges and presented them to the officer. As usual, he studied each carefully, handing Lee W.'s back.

"Her shoes are not appropriate." Officer Camden handed Dana's I/D back to her pointing at her shoes.

Dana stepped forward and politely wondered aloud? "My shoes, what do you mean?"

"Have you ever run in those shoes," was the officer's reply.

"Run? Well, no…not in these exact shoes."

"I suggest you change them, ma'am."

The two urologists looked at one another. Dana examined Lee W.'s boots, and then studied her low heeled black shoes. She looked back at the officer. "You think I may need to run?"

"Never know, Ma'am."

Lee W. stepped forward. "Look she has dressed appropriately! We have a patient, that is an inmate, to see."

Dana put her hand on Lee W.'s arm. "It's okay yaw-all. He's right; I have a pair of tennis shoes in my locker."

Dana took a moment to hurry back to the nurse's locker room in the OR. She returned, as Lee W. waited, in sensible white

Reeboks with pink laces. She would never visit the TDCJ again without them.

They were then buzzed in, the door closing with a click of finality.

Mr. Sampson was busy eating, what seemed to be a late breakfast when they entered. The inmate chewed grits loudly, with an open mouth, as the two walked across his room. He looked exclusively at Dana, continuing to masticate, eyeing first her face and then slowly down her body even to her feet. When he saw her shoes, he laughed quietly to himself. The two stood at the foot of his bed as the man washed down his chow with a swallow of hospital coffee.

"Mr. Sampson, how are you this morning?" Dana broke the silence and moved to check the man's catheter bag hanging by his right side, kneeling.

Sampson looked at the top of the woman's head as she bent down. He then looked up at Lee W. and smiled a gold-toothed smile.

"Are you okay, Mr. Sampson," she said now standing next to Lee W. at the foot of the bed.

"I hurt," he said still with a smile, the light blue eyes fixed on Dana.

"You shouldn't hurt anymore; do yaw-all mean the tube hurts?" Dana moved again to the man's side and lightly pushed on the tube's insertion site in his flank. The man winced at the pressure. The tube would relieve the severe kidney stone pain but often leave a lingering discomfort in the skin and muscles.

Sampson shook his head yes, again a gold tooth smirk on his face.

"You can take pain pills every four to six hours Mr. Sampson. Yaw-all should just ask the nurses. Now tomorrow, if you are alright with this, we're going to take you to the operating room. They'll put you to sleep, and we'll try to take that stone out through the bladder without an incision." Dana went on to explain the risks of the procedure which included infection, bleeding, and lethal type complications like heart attack, stroke, pneumonia, and blood clots. "If we cannot get the stone out through the bladder we'll make an incision and take the stone out like they did in Conroe."

With the mention of Conroe, the smile disappeared. "They took my kidney out in Conroe!"

With the mention of the kidney, Dana had to force herself not to say anything. She wanted to agree with the man and say that the surgery was unfortunate. "Yes…but… that was then, and you only have the right kidney, we need to take care of the stone carefully."

Sampson looked over at Lee W., who until now was silent. "Hey Chief, what's yaw-all got to say?"

Lee W. smiled. "Well I concur with Doctor Rausch, she will be doing the surgery I will be assisting her. Do you have any questions?"

"Ya assisting." For the first time, the man smiled a sincere smile. "Ya assisting, I like that Chief!"

Chapter 8

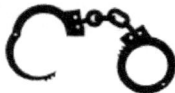

They did the Sampson case first thing in the morning. Lee W. and Dana scrubbed in the ancient porcelain sink, a 10-minute wash for this first case of the day. Dressed in a green scubsuit, Dana's wore white Reeboks with pink shoelaces. Her ponytail was pinned to the top of her head and covered with a large stretchy bouffant type surgery hat. Lee W's attire included scrubs, a tie-back surgical hat, and buffalo skin cowboy boots. Both surgeons wore leaded aprons to protect from x-rays.

"Did you get a KUB before he went to sleep?" Lee W. referred to the time-honored ritual of an x-ray done on the operating table before the stone patient goes to sleep. Why do you say? Stones are slippery creatures, and many have moved during the induction of anesthesia changing surgical plans drastically.

"Yes, the stone is still in the mid-ureter." She paused while scrubbing asking a teaching point of her attending. "Lee W., I have to tell you that I always think of cutting corners, though, have you ever seen a case where the x-ray made a difference?"

"Oh, never risk it, Dana. Here is a good case to prove that. One time I had a patient with a stone in the upper left ureter, unmoving for three to four weeks. After he was placed on the operating table, the x-rays showed the stone descended to the bladder. And that wasn't the worst finding."

"What else did you see?"

"Yaw-all I was prepared to place him in a flank position, make a 12th rib flank incision, and do an upper ureteralithotomy on the left. Not only had the left stone dropped into the bladder but he had formed a new stone now in the right ureter! No Dana, always get an x-ray before putting the man to sleep. It will save you from an embarrassing mistake one day."

"Oh what a disaster Lee W. I will remember that case, always go the extra mile and do a pre-operative film."

The two surgeons finished their scrub, shook their hands-free of water and soap, and backed into the operating room through the swinging door. Sampson was asleep, his legs up in stirrups. They draped the patient and began.

A ureteroscope is an 11 millimeter in diameter telescope 64 centimeters in length. Dana took the instrument and under vision placed the tip of the scope through the urethra and into the bladder. A balloon catheter was then placed through the scope and up the right ureter. Here the intramural ureter, which is the lowermost ureter that travels in the wall of the bladder was dilated. She then placed the tip of the ureteroscope into the ureteral opening and pushed the scope carefully under vision to the area of the mid-ureteral stone. Through the scope, a basket catheter was used to capture the stone and back it out dropping it in the bladder.

The procedure went like a textbook, using 18 minutes of anesthesia time from beginning to retrieving the stone from the bladder. X-ray documented that the stone was gone. Dye injected into his right nephrostomy tube showed good flow into the bladder and no injury to the ureter.

That afternoon Lee W. and Dana rounded over at the TDCJ together.

Officer Camden was on duty. After checking the badges, he gave silent approval to Dana's choice in shoes with a slight nod of his head.

The inmate was sleeping soundly when they entered his room. Dana knelt and checked his nephrostomy urine bag finding it draining well and pink that is only slightly blood tinged. She stepped back to the foot of the bed.

"I think we can turn off his nephrostomy tube in the morning." Here she indicated that in the morning they would turn the two-way valve on the tube off, diverting the urine down the ureter to the bladder. "If he does okay, then we can take the tube out the following day, and he can go on his way."

"Sounds okay, but I would watch him here a full day after the tube comes out. Yaw-all knows where he's going back to." Lee W. was concerned with sending the man back to Huntsville prematurely. The last thing he wanted was for him to have problems and have to return.

Sampson opened his eyes. He made eye-contact first with Lee W., and then with Dana. She waved and held up the plastic container with his stone.

"Where's my incision?" The patient was groggy, but as a matter of protocol, the stone must be visualized by the patient.

"No incision! We were lucky enough to get the stone out through the bladder. Again she shook the stone in the container and tried to show it to the inmate.

He then shuffled himself sitting upright. He examined his flank and right side, no incision. Sampson lay his head back and smiled almost a decent gold-toothed smile.

The next morning the TDCJ nurses turned the nephrostomy tube to off. Subsequently, he began urinating normally with no pain. The following day he was voiding well, had stable kidney function, and Dana removed the nephrostomy tube. He was discharged back to Huntsville the following day.

Sampson was transported to his "apartment" that night. The death row offenders live in single person, 60-square-foot cells, with each cell having a slit window and a concrete door. He backed up to the door, dropped to his knees, and extend his hands back through the narrow slot. The guard unhandcuffed him. He soon received his night meal through bean slots, gates in the cell doors. The meal consisted of grits and stew. The air was hot, kept at 85 degrees

Fahrenheit much to the prisoner's dislike. Death row inmates are not allowed to work. Theirs is a life of tedious boredom. When taken from his cell, an offender is strip searched. Then he stands, turns around, and waits for the door to be opened. The whole process of dropping to the knees and extending the arms backward is particularly challenging and painful for the older convicts with arthritis. Offenders receive individual recreation in a caged area. Depending on the custody level, death row offenders may be eligible for having radios. Death row inmates wear white jumpsuits, and the death row uniforms have the letters "DR" in black on the backs. The philosophy seems to be: "we keep you kenneled until your date."

Sampson ate his meal silently, leaving a good deal behind. He slid the finished tray through the bean slots and tapped the bars with his cup. "Done boss."
He lay on his cot and slept.

He awoke with another episode of right renal colic. The pain was incredible, on the right flank, with referral to the right groin. It shook him to the core, and he ended up in a huddle in the corner, perspiring. "Boss, I hurts again," he said after standing and yelling through the bean slot in his door.

When he started vomiting the guards moved the inmate to medical. Bobbie started him on a bucket watch, this time drawing labs to check his kidney function, potassium, and uric acid. He also contacted Dr. Wilson who saw the patient.

"I needs morph, Bobbie!" The patient's face was wet with perspiration, and he had a wild-eyed frightened look. The patient suffered from renal colic, medicine's worst type of pain. In comparing childbirth to renal colic, the latter is felt to be a worse pain. The morphine does not take the pain away but rather convinces the brain to not think about it. It was a long time waiting, but the dose was well received when administered.

Doctor Wilson entered the medical unit. He took one look at Sampson and knew the diagnosis. He had x-ray do a limited IVP, or an intravenous pyelogram, an x-ray with dye and X-rays.

"He has a right-sided stone, about 5 millimeters in size in the upper ureter Bobbie. Has he voided?"

"No, he hasn't voided since he arrived on medical."

"Put a catheter in, and get stat lytes and creatinine and uric acid."

Bobbie placed a small rubber tube in the bladder and found a small amount of bloody urine. He returned with the labs.

Wilson read the labs, creatinine up to 2.2 potassium up to 6.0 and uric acid 9.0.all abnormally elevated from the obstructed solitary right kidney. The Doctor ordered an ampule of D50W and an ampule of insulin IV. Here the glucose and insulin force the potassium into the cell and reduce the blood level of the potassium hoping to stop another seizure.

The next morning x-ray showed the stone had not moved. His creatinine was up to 3.1 the potassium 5.7. Dr. Wilson made rounds and examined the patient. Sampson was still in constant agony, taking pain med shots around the clock. The stone had not moved, and his labs were deteriorating. In addition, unlike prior stone episodes, the patient had a 101.3-degree fever.

"Mr. Sampson, yaw-all are going to have to go back to UTMB." Wilson pulled the patient's gown up and pointed to the high part of the abdomen. "Your stone is right about here and not moving. Your kidney function is deteriorating. I am very concerned about your fever as well."

Sampson said nothing, just closed his eyes as he suffered.

Chapter 9

The ride south to Galveston was not comfortable for the inmate. The right colicky pain and vomiting continued. He received a pain medicine injection upon leaving the prison medical ward but was forced to wait the two and a half hours for more until getting to Galveston. The transfer was in an old rickety ambulance whose shock absorbers had seen better days.

"Can't we get us a better ride here?" Sampson screamed out as they crashed over a particularly rough segment of road. It was the last thing he said on the trip south. He vomited again, the gray metal bucket now full, shaking over the top to the floor as he became silent.

"Did you notice that Sampson is not speaking?" One nurse said to the other.

"Take his vital signs." They found a temperature of 102 and blood pressure of 110 over seventy; his pulse elevated at 110 beats per minute, his respiration elevated at 25 breaths per minute.

One nurse picked up the receiver of the Citizens Band (CB) radio and called UTMB. "I have to talk to Doctor Upham of Urology," the male nurse said. After some time the doctor spoke on the CB.

"This is Doctor Mark Upham."

"Doctor, this is nurse Morris. I am monitoring inmate Sampson on his hospital ride south to Galveston and am concerned about him. He has a 102 fever, low blood pressure, elevated pulse and respiratory rate. He is unconscious; we can wake him but only temporarily."

"Can you draw a blood culture?"

"Yes, we have the equipment."

"Then draw a blood culture and a sample from the Foley catheter for culture. Place both in the refrigerator."

"There isn't much urine in the catheter, but I'll get a small sample and put it in a sterile cup."

"Then I want you to give him one gram of ampicillin and 80 mg of gentamycin IV after the cultures and a 10 grain rectal Tylenol suppository. Do you have those supplies?" Here he ordered two antibiotics, ampicillin, and gentamycin, and a Tylenol suppository for the fever.

"Yes, Doctor we do. I am going to go silent now and complete those orders."

They arrived at TDCJ around midnight, the old ambulance backing up to the loading dock in the back of the facility with horn rhythmically honking. Floodlights were on and lighted their way. Mark Upham stood on the loading dock looking down at the spectacle. He had so much to do that night; history and physical admission exams, emergency room, consult as well as other work, but Mr. Sampson would take priority. Correctional officers and the nurses exited the vehicle, opened the tailgate and wheeled Sampson on a gurney into the back of the hospital.

As the officers, did this Upham took the opportunity to look at the man, sweating and grimacing not aware of his surroundings.

Dressed as a death row inmate with a white button-down shirt with an open collar and DR stenciled in black on the back. He wore white matching pants, the right leg significantly shorter than the left, worn over orange shower shoes.

"He doesn't look so good," the intern said to whoever would listen. The men wheeled the inmate into the hospital with little attention, down the hall, and into the same empty room that he resided in before. They lifted the man off the gurney and onto his hospital bed dropping him with a bolt on an empty flimsy mattress.

"Get vital signs as soon as you can," Upham said to the male nurse who met them.

"Doctor, his oral temperature is 102.3, his blood pressure 100 over sixty, his respiratory rate is 30 breaths per minute."

Upham recalled the man's blood pressure on his prior admission running in the 130's, a significant decline. He did a quick physical and noted a sweaty male who responded only when shook awake. He called Dana on the phone: "must be totally obstructed again, and with the fever, I don't know, I am worried about him."

"I agree, we need to have x-ray put a perc in that kidney, but anesthesia will have to watch him during the procedure." Dana and

Upham were concerned over the man because he had an obstructed solitary kidney with a fever. This implied pyonephrosis, a pus-filled obstructed kidney which can lead to sepsis, shock, and irreparable damage to the kidney. The treatment is, once again, drain the kidney's urine with a tube through the skin and kidney.

Upham moved to a phone and called the anesthesiologist on call. He explained the case in detail. The anesthesiologist was very busy and reluctant to help. He soon realized the risks, however, and hesitantly agreed to stand by and monitor Sampson during the procedure.

Dr. Chad Finklestein placed a tube through the skin and kidney leaving the tube to gravity, that is sitting on the floor. Upon entering the kidney, he found gray foul pus under pressure. During the procedure, the patient's blood pressure dropped, and they had to place the inmate in Trendelenburg position, legs up raising the blood pressure. He then became stable, and they brought the man back to his hospital bed in TDJC.

It was incredible how quickly the inmate recovered.

Dana made rounds at the TDCJ that morning by herself. She would never do that again. She passed the two guards sitting in gray metal chairs, with a smile, and entered the room. She found the man sitting up in his bed eating his breakfast happily. He was bare-chested, his eagle tattoo visible for all the world to see. In his right side was the nephrostomy tube, draining relatively clear urine to a bag on the floor.

"Mr. Sampson, you look so much better!"

Sampson looked up from his tray with a mouth full, eggs falling from his lips, his golden teeth flashing. He looked at the woman silently, as a predator, setting his plastic fork down and saying nothing.

Dana stood with her arms crossed expecting some discourse. Sampson was silent, so she moved to the right side of the bed and kneeled, looking at the urine bag. The man threw his tray across his body, grabbed his right pant leg tearing the cuff to reveal a crudely made knife or shank. He grabbed her ponytail and put the razor-sharp blade to her throat. He stood pulling the woman in front of himself.

One of the officers fell off his chair, the other stood and drew his gun.

"What yaw-all is doing Sampson? Put the blade down and let the girl go."

Sampson had no intention of giving up his hostage. He drug her across the room to a large handicapped sized bathroom and bolt locked the door.

"You and me are going to get to know each other, Dana! I'm a *killa*, remember!"

Dana fought like a banshee, pulling away from the man. She turned and kneed him in the groin.

Her actions just seemed to increase the man's excitement. He fought with his weapon at her throat and brought her down to sit on the floor in front of him. Sampson forced his mouth on hers. She bit his tongue. "You bitch," he said spitting out blood. "You're gonna take this and like it," Sampson said as he tried to press up against her.

The officers banged on the locked door. One turned and went for help in the hallway. Alarms sounded throughout the area, mayhem beginning on the ward.

"We're gonna have some fun now Dana." He threw the woman down in front of him with the collar of her white coat and sat on her all the while holding the blade to her throat.

Soon the hospital room filled with multiple gun-toting officers. There was chaos, yelling, screaming, lights flipped on, several banging on the door. One pried the door with a crowbar and violently threw the door open, a bevy of officers then filling the bathroom toting guns and yelling. One grabbed Sampson by the hair and threw him off the girl, the blade shooting harmlessly across the floor. Soon three officers sat on top of the man.

Dana stood slowly, moving to the corner holding her neck. She scooted along the wall, bent and picked up the blade. She stood looking at the scene as the officers secured the man, and then quickly moved into the hospital room. Her coat was ripped open, her scrub suit top nearly pulled off, her ponytail pulled up over her head. She straightened her jacket and repositioned her hair. She walked slowly out of the room and sat with a crash on the officer's gray metal chair.

Dana tried to calm herself. She sat staring at the floor as she slowed her breathing. Dana looked down at the shank in her right hand. What she found was made from a butter knife, approximately five inches in length and drawn to a point, one edge sharpened.

They secured Sampson, his arms bound with cuffs behind him in a violent scuffle with a houseful of officers. They lifted him off the floor, pulled him out the door past the woman down the hall and threw him into a locked cell.

As the man passed, Dana looked at his face without fear. Sampson smiled an open-mouthed, golden tooth smile but would not make eye-contact.

Chapter 10

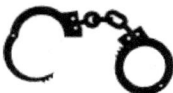

Abbott T. Frankenstein, MD, as with his namesake, was a hulking tower of a man. He stood just over six foot seven, dressed in his usual 58 extra-long Italian tailored suit, a flat-top recently trimmed without wings, and black polished wing-tipped shoes. He looked distantly out of the full-length window that made up the majority of the wall of his fifth-floor office and over his kingdom, the sprawling campus of UTMB.

He had reason to look proudly, for he built the campus through his now eleven-year tenure as president of the state's first university medical center. This morning, though, he was troubled as he gazed, for the Governor had just called him, he too unhappy at the course of their troubled patient, Billie James Sampson.

Politically Von Mitchell, the first term governor of the state of Texas, was a practical man, especially on crime associated subjects. His campaign vowed to execute the country's most heinous criminals, and the way it was going with Sampson, execution would be a very distant event if ever.

The man's incarceration was bogged down with surgery after surgery for kidney stones rather than punishing custody. A surgeon, with no business practicing medicine, removed a perfectly intact kidney, he had a grand-mal seizure while interned in the medical unit, and now he had violently assaulted a female physician, a chief resident of this institution. Yes, the governor's phone call was not a pleasant one, insisting that something was finally done with Mr. Sampson. The question was what?

"Doctor. Frankenstein? Doctor's Hickok and Rausch are here to see you," his timid secretary, Suzie announced electronically over the newly installed intercom. Frankenstein took a moment to refresh his antacid level, taking a swig of Maalox from an oversized bottle he kept hidden in his desk, careful to wipe his lips of the chalky substance with his breast pocket handkerchief. He then buzzed back to the woman to escort the two into his office, as he stood just inside the mahogany double door waiting for the two physicians.

Doctor Hickok entered first dressed in a white coat over a pale green button-down collar shirt, with a green and white striped tie, and black trousers over a polished pair of black buffalo hide cowboy boots. Doctor Rausch followed dressed as well in a white coat over a modest beige dress, and interestingly white rebook tennis shoes with pink laces. The three exchanged pleasantries and handshakes. The two urologists sat on the white flowered couch while Frankenstein pulled up an ox-blood overstuffed chair.

With a little knock, Suzie entered carrying a tray with Grandma Rae's black tea blend from the panhandle of Texas in a Chinese porcelain pot and matching cups. She poured each a cup adding sugar to their liking.

"Lee W., tell me about the status of Mr. Sampson." Frankenstein got right to the point, holding a cup of tea in his huge hand and sipping.

"Well, he was admitted with right pyonephrosis. This was secondary to a stone in the upper right ureter with complete obstruction and pus above the stone in the kidney."

"Let me stop you right there, how did he get the infection?" Frankenstein placed his teacup down on the table and looked with curiosity at the two.

"He has been instrumented here at UTMB and experience shows, even with the judicial use of antibiotics, that post instrumentation infections occur."

"Okay, we probably gave him that infection, is that what you are trying to say?"

"Well, yaw-all, I don't really like those terms, but yes, he probably was infected during one of our procedures. It is a risk of instrumentation, Abbott. On the other hand, he may have gotten a urinary tract infection at the Wall's, it is impossible to say."

"Okay, I agree, it doesn't matter, please continue." Frankenstein sat back in the leather chair listening.

" Let's see, where was I? Yes, he had pyonephrosis with impending sepsis and low blood pressure, and a percutaneous nephrostomy tube was placed in the kidney by interventional radiology. Upon entering the kidney, pus under pressure was found. Since then, with drainage, he has had a rapid improvement with correction of his renal failure, resolution of his fever, and improvement in his mental status."

"What bacteria did he grow from that kidney?"

"E. coli, just an ordinary urinary tract bacteria."

"Well, you say improvement, that's to say improvement to the point of assault, Lee W.? Dana, how are you after this predator got ahold of you?"

Dana put her teacup down. She placed her hand on her right neck self-consciously covering what had become a deep bruise. "Well, Doctor Frankenstein, I am fine, this animal is not going to stop me."

Frankenstein looked at her shoes. "I notice you wear running shoes Dana, is that to get away from this disgusting excuse for a human?"

Frankenstein's language surprised Dana, but she agreed totally with his words. "Yes, for a matter of fact, I have been wearing these whenever I go to the TDCJ with the security officer's direction. I had them on that day, however, and he still got me alone in a bathroom."

"We are so sorry for that attack, Dana. The University apologizes to you as do I. Would you like to press charges; I could refer you to a university lawyer."

"I am okay, Doctor Frankenstein. I would really like to just move on. Chalk it up to experience, that animal will never prey on me again. Thanks for the lawyer but let's just roll past that event."

"You feel physically fine then?"

"Yes," Dana said scooting back on the couch and uncovering her bruise by removing her hand.

"How are you mentally, dear?"

"I am fine…I'm fine Doctor Frankenstein."

"Well, I am not sure you should be treating the man anymore. Lee W., what is your thought?"

Dana spoke up instantly. "Sir, if I may speak, I will not let this killer win. I request to continue my job as chief resident, and that includes even taking care of Billie James Sampson. I can't let him win!"

"Yes, Dana and I have talked about this, Abbott. She is adamant about continuing to take care of the inmate. She is very brave and extremely tough. But I have to agree with her. It is her call in my mind." Lee W. took a sip of the tea and then set the cup on the coffee table.

"Okay," Frankenstein said. "Dana be cautious, but continue to carry on your duties with this monster. I am meeting with Officer Thomas and Bill Rapport the staff sergeant of the TDCJ and the chief medical commander of the TDCJ will institute new security measures to inhibit his freedoms."

"Are we facing admissions every few weeks with renal colic and failure, with surgeries every few weeks?" Frankenstein stood as he asked this, straightening his back.

"Well as his medullary sponge kidney is active, yes it seems that he drops a stone down every week or so. When he does, that is a solitary kidney, and so it becomes significant with the risk of acute renal failure."

"Is there anything medically that can reduce this frequency?" Frankenstein enquired?

"Not really, other than drinking massive amounts of water which we have encouraged. MSK is somewhat different in that it is a congenital abnormality where the tubules in the kidney have swollen areas that collect urine and form stones. Then it is just a matter of time before the stone drops down." Lee W. stood as well and moved to stand next to Frankenstein.

"He's most likely going to continue to make these stones then, and then drop them down and obstruct the ureter. Great…were in for admission after admission." Frankenstein said with some frustration.

Dana spoke up. "Lee W. was telling me about an ileal ureter."

"What is an ileal ureter?" Frankenstein wondered?

Lee W. moved to a blackboard across the room. "I'll draw a picture for you, Abbott. "On the blackboard, he drew a right kidney with a renal pelvis or funnel and ureter or tube connecting to the bladder. He placed a density in the upper ureter representing the stone that Sampson had. "In an ileal ureter, you take a loop of ileum generally based on the ileocolic artery." Here he referred to removing a segment of bowel for the procedure. "The length will be measured intraoperatively, but generally is about 60 centimeters or so. The loop of bowel is turned 180 degrees, so an iso-peristaltic segment is hooked first to the renal pelvis and the other end to the dome of the bladder." Here he referred to the need to have the direction of the bowel movement or peristalsis from the kidney to bladder or so-called iso-peristaltic. The proximal end of the loop is sewn to the renal pelvis, the distal end to the dome of the bladder. "All visible stones would be removed including the one in the right ureter, but the ureter is left intact.

"The idea is to replace the very narrow ureter where a stone is continually lodging with a very wide loop of the bowel where the stones can just move on through. This would allow him to pass stones whenever, without obstruction and episodes of renal colic or renal failure."

Frankenstein was very interested in this solution. He moved to the blackboard and began to ask questions. "Is this a big operation?"

"Yes, quite large and lengthy, but really gets the man back to the Wall's unit and allows him to live a life without episodes of kidney stones problems. The patient's pass a great deal of mucus in their urine, but they get used to that."

"What about absorption, does the bowel absorb the urine?" Frankenstein wondered whether such a long segment of bowel might reabsorb the urine and create metabolic problems.

Lee W. smiled, he realized the internist thinking here. "With people with good renal function, and Sampson's baseline creatinine is 0.8 mg per deciliter which is quite good, the urine absorption is handled by the kidneys and no adverse effect is noted."

"Where is this operation generally used, Lee W.?"

"Dana spoke up. I did a review article on that subject Doctor Frankenstein. The majority ileal-ureters were performed for damaged ureters with a stricture and ureteral fistulas. A smaller number was for recurrent episodes of renal colic like our patient, but a 91% success rate was noted overall."

"Quite good," Frankenstein said.

Lee W. continued. "Yes, this actually answers the problem that Sampson has perfectly. We cannot control his stone passage rate; it seems to be quite high. When he does pass a stone, he is often in kidney failure. What happens is an emergent visit to UTMB, with all the manpower and risks to staff. If the ureteral-substitution, which is essentially what the ileal ureter is, works, he can pass stones whenever with no pain and no obstruction. A date with the gallows would be in his future then, which is what the Governor wants I guess."

"I am quite excited," the president said. "Prepare this piece of trash for surgery and get going on the procedure!"

Chapter 11

The man sat squarely, and with a sense of grandeur, at the carved oaken desk, surrounded by decorated walls, sculpture, and paintings. He silently removed a key from his jetted suit pocket, turned slowly, and opened the desk's top side drawer. Within was a black leather embroidered leather box with a mirrored interior, which he set carefully before him, with mounting anticipation and desire. It was filled with white magic powder, and he took a small golden spoon and snorted a pile, first in the left and then the right nostril with such a thrill. Throwing back in the chair he shook his head for a short time with his eyes tightly closed and watering. He then wiped his face with his handkerchief and placed a finger on his gum and rubbed. He replaced the box and placed the key back in his pocket.

Bounding up from his desk he moved with a strident pace, opened a beautifully molded side door and entered the chamber.

"Gentlemen I am sorry to keep yaw-al waiting." He shook each's hand who then introduced themselves.

"Governor, I am Luther Jackson. It is a great honor to meet you." Said a tall black man with a cornrow hairstyle.

"Governor, I am Felix Artain, glad to meet you." Said a shorter white, balding man with thick black glasses.

"So, glad to meet you, Governor, I am Doctor J.D. Wilson from Conroe Texas." He was a tall, thin set man with a red-brown hair and a bushy mustache.

"Gentlemen have a seat," the Governor said asking the three to sit on the flowery embroidered couch in his office's sitting area. "Do yaw-all want coffee or Tea?"

Everyone indicated coffee. The Governor pushed a button on the coffee table and spoke to his secretary. "Bring us a pot of coffee Judy if you will."

"What is it that I can help you with today?" The Governor asked. He was a thin blond haired man with long bushy sideburns. He was dressed in a finely tailored gray suit with a red white and blue bowtie with a matching hanky.

Luther Jackson spoke for the group. "The first subject that we would like to discuss is freedom. We, Felix and I, represent a citizen of Texas namely Billie James Sampson. He is unfortunately incarcerated in Huntsville, an innocent victim of the judicial system, held wrongly for first-degree murder facing execution. As you may be aware, he has suffered at the hands of the medical system even to the point of losing a perfect kidney to the malpractice of one Doctor James "Slim" McCormack."

Felix Artain then continued. "We are here to encourage a pardon of this tragic man."

The Governor grimaced at the mention of pardon. He shook his head slowly negatively.

Artain went on. "His medical condition is such that the medical system surrounding him is inferior, and continually mistreating him. Case in point, "Slim" McCormack who has removed, if you can believe it, a perfectly normal kidney."

The Governor stepped right in. "This man is a killer, councilors, we get no place beginning with this outrageous request for pardon. There will not be a pardon."

"We know that you would not do so today, but Governor we have a written appeal and would like to leave it with you, for your future consideration." Jackson removed a bound volume from his leather briefcase and handed it to the Governor. The Governor set the tome down on the coffee table without looking at it.

"Just so you understand my opposition to this pardon from the get-go."

Judy entered through the door knocking lightly. She set down a china serving tray, cups, and pot of hot Texas grown coffee and began pouring for the visitors. "Will you have cream and or sugar?" was asked of each.

"Please Governor, keep an open mind on this gentleman's innocence, and if you will we could go on to discuss the malpractice issue."

"Please do, "the governor said after wiping his brow with his hanky

Doctor J.D. Wilson spoke up. "I can attest to the malpractice committed. Mr. Sampson has kidney stone disease. He now is in the difficult situation where he has just a right kidney which he recurrently obstructs and goes into kidney failure. He had a seizure because of this while I was attending him."

"Yes, I understand the situation, what can we do at this point?"

"Withdraw James "Slim" McCormack's medical license, causing him to stop practicing this inferior brand of medicine. We will leave the disposition of the inmate's medical condition to the UTMB urologist for the time being."

A knock occurred on the side door. The Governor stood and opened it. A young short-ish black woman with a moderate, neatly trimmed afro hairstyle, dressed in a navy-blue suit and heels entered. "Governor I am so sorry to be late, I couldn't get away from the court. I am Rita Blackwell, and I am Doctor McCormack's lawyer."

"Councilor, what say you concerning the medical license of Doctor McCormack?" The Governor wondered.

"Dr. McCormack is a fine tenured physician. He has never been involved in any malpractice litigation, his record is exemplary. He has no complaints lodged with the medical board."

"These fine gentlemen," the Governor said pointing to the three men. "These two lawyers and one physician are making the case that his medical license should be revoked based on his care of Mr. Billie James Sampson."

"Of course, Doctor McCormack should continue to be licensed. He has served the state well; Mr. Sampson is not the only charity case from Huntsville that the good Doctor has taken care of, and always pro bono I should add."

Artain stood from the couch, coffee cup in hand. "The issue is Mr. Sampson's loss of a perfectly good kidney which has relegated him to the situation that he is in now. Why did the good Doctor remove that kidney?"

Blackwell stood and addressed the man. "During Sampson's 28 years of life, he passed nearly hundreds of left-sided kidney stones. Doctor McCormack removed three stones in a three-month period. The removal of the left kidney treated the acute problem."

"The removal of the left kidney made stones in the right kidney acute medical emergencies, with acute kidney failure," Jackson responded.

"Proper consent was obtained; the patient knew the risks involved and agreed to the surgery." She turned to the Governor asking for relief. "I feel I'm two-timed here, Sir."

"You are the counselor, and really triple teamed for the Doctor is supporting the removal of his license as well. Let me step in here. First of all, the reason for this meeting for me is that I want this animal, and excuse me councilors that is what he is, I want this inmate executed. I based my election to this office on tough criminal prosecution and using the death penalty vigorously. That is what the people of Texas want, it is what I want. Now, to that end, I have nothing to do with the license of Slim McCormack. That is an issue for the medical board. Now you three arguing with the nice counselor does not change my opinion. I will make a statement to the medical board after reviewing all your materials. My opinion, however, caries little weight I am afraid, with the Texas medical board."

"Now, yaw-all, I don't want to read about our meeting especially the kidney issue in the media. Please do not reveal the details of this issue." With that the Governor ushered the lawyers and doctor to the side door, ending the conversation. A return to his office was needed.

```
https://tsw.createspace.com/title/8250025/review
https://tsw.createspace.com/title/8250025/review
https://tsw.createspace.com/title/8250025/review
```

https://tsw.createspace.com/title/8250025/review
https://tsw.createspace.com/title/8250025/review

She was there when Lee W. and Dana returned from the meeting with Frankenstein, standing at the elevator door as it opened as nice as pie.

"Doctor Hickok."

"Hello, Jennifer."

"I'm off for the OR Lee W.," Dana said moving off quickly.

Lee W. and Jennifer Harry talked as they walked down the hall towards Lee W's office. "What can you tell me about the assault on Doctor Rausch by Billie Sampson?"

"I can tell you nothing."

"Are you saying the assault did not occur?"

"I am answering no comment, Jennifer."

"I know through other sources that the assault occurred, is Doctor Rausch off the case of Billie Sampson?"

"That I can refute, she is Sampson's physician."

"What was the extent of the injury."

"No comment."

"I hear of a big surgery to correct his problem. Can you give me details on this?"

Lee W. stopped and looked at the reporter with scorn. "Jennifer, where did you get that piece of info?"

"My sources are my sources, and I cannot reveal them, Doctor Hickok."

"Then we are at our usual impasse."

Lee W. entered his office the reporter left down the hallway. He sat at his desk, thought about his Sweat Amber. Where were these media leaks coming from? He supposed the leak about the assault came from the TDCJ staff. But where did the leak about the ileal ureter? Some person in the Frankenstein's office, most certainly. It would be interesting to see tomorrow's Galveston Daily County News.

Chapter 12

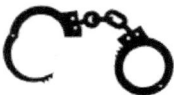

The surgery was over, everything accomplished as planned. Lee W., Dana, and the senior resident Duke McHugh performed a right ileal ureter and removed the stone, a ureteralithotomy. Here, after removal of the stone a 60 centimeter or so "loop" of small bowel called ileum was used to replace the right ureter. The idea then was to give a larger diameter route for stones to travel to the bladder, hence preventing obstruction and renal failure.

"All right, yaw-all I leave him to you." Lee W. said to Dana and Duke as he left the operating room.

"Duke, write post-op orders, let's start him on TPN (Total Parenteral Nutrition). Place the nephrostomy tube to gravity drainage, we'll leave the Jackson-Pratt drains to suction for now. Keep him on the pre-op antibiotics. Here she was prescribing TPN which is high caloric intravenous feeding. Tube-wise the right nephrostomy tube in place before surgery would be kept and drained to the floor. The several drains placed at surgery were so-called Jackson Pratt suction drains. "We will recover him in the TDCJ ICU for a few days. Make sure that the security team has a head's up and that they watch him like a hawk."

Dana reached to the instrument tray and retrieved the removed stone in a plastic container so that she could show it to the patient as was her practice. It would be quite a while before she could do so.

Billie James Sampson felt something that he had not felt in many years, fright. He was a petty thief since childhood, a violent felon later in life. The man fought his way through life, battling since he could remember. He fought for his living, paying more often than not in his own blood. He soon learned to beat women for his pastime, a much more cowardly way to avoid the unavoidable injury. It never really caught up with him, except at the end where he eventually paid with his freedom. But scared, he couldn't remember that feeling. Anger had clouded his eyes through the years. He used it to forget his past, his father, his childhood. Yes anger, but fright not really.

Dana's words had gotten to him. He could remember them nearly verbatim. Risks of the procedure, infection, bleeding, and then the word possible death. He had sat silently as the jury read his death penalty. He would eventually face the *needle*, but it was so far in the distant future that he did not feel the same gravity when he heard the jury foreman. Dana had gotten him, as he listened to her discussion of surgical risks he realized he could die and soon.

Chapter 13

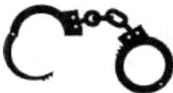

He lay on the hard operating table, a silly paper hat covering his head, oxygen blowing cold air into his nose. It was freezing in the white-walled room as the pre-med drug began to cloud his vision. The smell was antiseptic, and he wished with a panic that he could get up and walk out.

Billie James Sampson felt something absent in his mind for years, fright. He was a petty thief since childhood, a violent felon later. He fought his way through life, battling since he could remember. He fought for his living, paying more often than not in his own blood. He soon learned to beat women for his pastime, a much more cowardly way to avoid injury.

His violence never really caught up with him, except at the end where he paid with his freedom. But scared, he really could not remember the feeling. Anger clouded his eyes through the years.

He used it to forget his past, his father, his childhood. Yes anger, but fright not really.

Dana's words had gotten to him. He could remember them nearly verbatim now trembling, as he looked up at the huge operative lights. Risks of the procedure, infection, bleeding, and then the concept of possible death. He had sat silently in rage as the jury read his death penalty. He would eventually face the *needle,* something he knew he deserved. That date was so far in the distant future that he did not feel the same gravity when he heard the jury foreman. Dana had gotten him, as he listened to her discussion of surgical risks he realized he could die and soon. Her words now echoed in his rapidly sedated brain.

The face of the anesthesiologist looking at him from an upside-down perspective was the last thing he was sure about as the gas induced dream took hold.

The boy sat on the wooden floor believing, but more so hoping to be somewhere else the day it happened again. He was day-dreaming as usual, sadness clouding the edge of his thoughts as always. The summer heat was stifling, the humidity overwhelming, as it hung in the air of the rusting, filthy, double-wide. The crackling television set blared a blubberish scene of American gibberish from the front room. He knew that he was not safe, however, as whiskey and evil were awake again.

The fire red Mustang made an imaginary roar as it circled in front of him. It had wide rear tires, and he could hear them squealing. He saw one just like it, scurrying down the highway. It was etched in his memory, and he wondered with a lonesome thought whether he would one day drive one as well. He marked the car, his name Billie, carved in the roof of his toy.

He was beside him before he could run, the man looking down with a half-empty bottle in his left hand. The whiskey was the sign, safety was nowhere. The boy looked up at the man knowing what to expect, hoping he was wrong.

"Daddy!"

The old leather boot crushed the toy car and kicked it across the room. He hit him as always with his hand, a slap on the back of his head sending him across the floor sliding partway under the unmade twin bed. He was dazed, or he would have run, as the man latched on to the back of his belt. He tossed him across the bed like *a child's toy, and with his belt now in his hand, he thrashed him across his bare legs.*

The beating went on. It evolved into the man choking him with callused hands. His neck was crushed, and as he gagged, he could smell the grease left in the man's palms from hundreds of overhauls at the garage. He was behind the boy, and he pounded his face into the mattress repeatedly as he slowly tightened down on his neck. The pain was now overcoming him, his head throbbing like a firehouse bell, as he gasped for air.

He was unconscious when the true disrespect occurred. His pants were torn and pulled violently to the floor. The man huffing and puffing as he strained to his task. Yes, and it sickened him, the man always cried when he was done.

He awoke left now in that vulnerable position. Thrown over the edge of the unmade bed, his torn pants hung shamelessly down at his feet. The blood was always such a fright, and he gathered himself trying to hide it. The bruises would go away, no-one would say anything. When he got big enough the assaults ended with one last violent altercation where he beat his Father with his baseball bat. It amounted to his first arrest and prison time.

He was awake, at least he thought so. The dream was so real, one that he had quite often. Soon the pain in his belly was horrible, pulling, burning, and aching and he forgot the disturbing reverie. It began at the bottom of his ribcage and extended below his bellybutton. A hard tube was in his nose, and he could not breathe on his own. He noticed the rhythm of breaths being forced into his unready lungs, the jolt aggravating his abdominal pain.

A lovely nurse with a crisp white hat stood at his side. She pushed some medicine into and checked his IV. He glanced upwards; a yellow bottle dripping slowly into his neck. The color suggested to Billie James Sampson that they were infusing urine, in reality, it was TPN or Total Parental Nutrition colored yellow by the included vitamins.

The morphine brought some relief from the abdominal pain allowing him to accommodate the ventilator breaths. Soon he was dreaming away.

When he awoke, the man was sitting at the foot of the gurney, his skinny legs crossed daintily at the knee. He was dressed all in black, a white-skinned, smallish man with a sharp-toothed, accusatory smile and greasy black hair. When he noticed that Sampson was awake, he moved to his side, a long-nailed index finger tracing a cross on his bedsheets. The man looked at him directly, his eyes darkly highlighted by a thick line of red mascara. He grabbed the tube in his throat and shook it violently.

"Oh shit...," Sampson yelled out in silence only to himself. He violently coughed, launching a paroxysm of pain in his abdomen. He was intubated, an endotracheal tube filling his larynx and muzzling his voice. Panic coursed through him as he lay in paralyzed silence looking past the man for help. He lifted his leg hoping to flag someone down. No one responded.

The man stepped back and laughed a wicked laugh. He pushed back his black hair with a white long-nailed hand.

"My friend, I find you finally awake," the man said in a frightening horse whisper. He grabbed the tube, shook it bringing another paroxysmal cough to Sampson's tortured lungs. He threw back the bed sheet to reveal a long mid-line incision oozing drops of blood.

The man looked directly into the eyes of Sampson. He gestured theatrically with his hand. "See how they have left you!"

The man howled in demonic laughter, produced a glass syringe from his suit-jacket and injected it into his IV.

A horrible crushing pain flashed across Sampson's chest. The EKG's alarm began squealing, a paper tracing rolling out from the bedside machine. The nurse arrived at his side with fright in her eyes. She flipped a switch on the wall, "code blue ICU," repeatedly shouted overhead.

The room soon filled with a hysterical group of men and women. They dropped the head of his bed with a violent crash. Another raised the foot of the bed to the point of falling.

A man began chest percussions to a rapid beat. "One and two and three and four and five…" With each, he pushed down with crosslinked hands and crushing pressure over Sampson's sternum. A man at the head of the bed forced air down his endotracheal tube with a bag.

"Oh…Oh…Oh…" Sampson cried out in tortuous pain with each beat of forced silence, his legs bouncing.

A white coated woman at the foot of the bed yelled out orders, the nurse quickly infusing syringes full of drugs. "Stop CPR!"

A paper tracing was run off from the EKG. "Sinus rhythm," the woman yelled with excitement after viewing it. They stopped chest compressions and the room gradually emptied. The nurse slowly cranked the bed to a horizontal position.

The demon-man looked down from his position sitting in the corner, upon the wall-mounted television. He looked fulfilled, shook his head slowly; a sinister smile of satisfaction covering his lips.

☞

Dana heard the *code blue* overhead. She knew immediately what it represented. She ran to the TDCJ making it to Sampson's room as the chaos began. Anesthesia was at the head of the bed bagging air into his lungs interspersed with chest compressions. A man in green scrubs and a white coat was draped over Sampson's chest performing rhythmic chest percussions. Pharmacy stood at the foot of the bed with a large med-cart dispersing medications. The Medical Officer of the Day (MOD) was barking instructions.

"One and two and three and four and five…" CPR continued vigorously to the spoken rhythm.

"Give an amp of bicarb, 75 milligrams of lidocaine, and an amp of calcium carbonate. Can someone draw a blood gas?" A white coated man stepped to the side of the patient and drew an arterial sample of blood from his right femoral artery in the groin.

"Does anyone know this patient?" The MOD yelled to everyone in the room.

Dana moved alongside her. "He's Billie James Sampson. He's a 28-year-old black male death-row inmate. Just yesterday we performed a right ileal ureter for recurrent ureteral stones, he has a solitary right kidney with good renal function."

The MOD went on. "Well, we were called and found him in V-fib." Here she referred to a rapid abnormal heartbeat. "I am about to stop CPR and get a tracing. STOP CPR!"

The chest percussions stopped, and an EKG tracing whirred off. "We have sinus rhythm the MOD said to the group. "Do we have pulses?"

The arterial blood gas drawer felt for a pulse in the groin. "Yes, we do and quite strong."

"Fine, let's put him back in a horizontal position. Yaw-all can move out of here." The MOD grabbed Sampson's chart and began writing a "Code" note in the chart.

Dana moved slowly to the bedside. She looked up at the EKG which now was tracing out a normal sinus heart rhythm. Her eyes dropped to Sampson's. His were wide open, his blue eyes dreadful and wild looking. Tears coursed down his cheeks. Dana looked at the man with some fear in the back of her mind. She remembered her last encounter with the violent man. He was pitiful, though, terrified and shuttering. Slowly she picked up his hand and held it. She said: "You're alright now Mr. Sampson."

Chapter 14

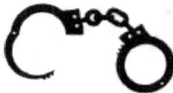

"I'll have a bourbon. A double!" Doctor James "Slim" McCormack spoke politely to the waiter as he slid into a black leathered backroomed booth of Shagshaw's Steak Restaurant. When the waiter returned with his beverage, he took a deep swallow and then touched the iced glass to his sweating brow.

Slim was nervous, meeting his half-brother for a "talk." Whenever these meetings were arranged, bad things generally resulted. He remembered his brother's insistence that Slim hire a young woman with no nursing experience. Slim knew she was trouble the moment he heard about her. Sure enough, her short two-week tenure ending in a sexual harassment suit was the result. Then there was their Mother, Barbra. She was a *piece of cake*, an aging alcoholic who was not doing well. His brother could afford to have her looked after. Slim wanted nothing to do with *Babs*. He signaled for a refill, using up time wondering the man's issue as he emptied a sugar packet onto the table.

An uprising at the front doors marked Von W. Mitchel's arrival, a slick-dressed man surrounded discreetly by Texas Ranger agents. The man just blew in surrounded by his personnel.

"Hi James," said the Texas governor sliding in across the table, wearing his usual red white and blue bowtie. He missed, perhaps on purpose, Slim's outstretched hand, as he turned to a beautiful assistant with a large mobile phone. "Yes? Not now," shaking his head and tossing around his long blond locks. "Take care of it."

"How are yaw-all?" The Governor said after handing the phone back to the woman. "Send that memo to Joshua, Joyce."

"I'm fine Von." Slim had no time for pleasantries. They were brothers by separate fathers, and he was never close to the powerful man. "What is it that you want?"

"In do time James," the Governor said with an annoyed look. "What's eating you?"

"I have a practice to run yaw-all. You blow in from Austin with your entourage. Probably a private plane fueled on the tarmac and funded by our treasury. Yaw-all, I never eat this early in the afternoon."

"Yes." The woman handed the Governor a paper which he signed without looking at it.

A male waiter arrived nervously interrupting them with a well-scrubbed smile. He introduced himself and gave each a leather menu for their perusal. "Today's special is the Chilean Seabass," he said with a grin.

"The rib-eye. Well done," Slim said handing back the menu without opening it eyeing the Governor the entire time.

"What about a potato sir?"

"What?...Yeah, a baked potato with just butter is fine."

"And you sir," the waiter said turning to the Governor.

"The bass. You said it was Chilean?"

"Yes, fresh in today. It is sautéed in a garlic and lemon sauce with fresh capers. It comes with mixed vegetables. How about a potato for you?"

"No, I'm fine son…Oh, an incredibly dry vodka martini with two olives." The Governor said handing back the menu.

A silent pause ensued as the two brothers stared at each other.

"Come on Von, you didn't come here for Chilean Sea Bass cooked with capers." Slim sat back in the booth. Nerves passed from the man as the alcohol took root. He finished his second bourbon with a deep swig.

The martini arrived, and the Governor took a small sip. He looked up at Slim with a tight-faced smile. "How's Lucille? How are the kids?"

"They're fine. Get to the point!"

The Governor wet his lips with his tongue. He stared at Slim for some time. "What can you tell me about Billie…James Sampson?"

"Who?"

"Come on, you know who I'm talking about. That criminal, that dirtbag. You know…death row? Remember? You took his kidney out."

Slim looked down and picked up an imaginary piece of lint off the table. He wished he still smoked, thinking to himself how he would blow smoke profusely into the Governor's face. This was

Von W. Mitchel at his noisy best. Yes, he knew the patient's name and the case backward and forwards. He knew that he had left-sided medullary sponge kidney and that the treatment was to remove the left kidney. He did not know what had happened since the surgery, however. Slim realized that he was going to find out. "Mr. Sampson, yes I am aware of him."

The waiter returned with their dishes and with fanfare placed them before the two customers. "Watch out now, these plates are incredibly hot. Would you care for ground pepper?"

Slim shook his head negatively all the while looking at the Governor.

"Yes, definitely," said the Governor.

Both men took bites of their dishes. "Oh, the bass is delicious," the Governor said picking up his martini for a sip. He took one olive and popped it into his mouth. "Your steak looks positively burnt. I have never known why you insist on a well-done Texas steak? It ruins the taste, James!"

At this point, a short, portly man with an elaborate combover stood in front of the two. "Hello Governor, my name is Jack Shagshaw, the owner of this establishment."

"Yes, John I've met you before." Gesturing at Slim, he went on. "This is my brother, Jack. Doctor James McCormack from Conroe, a very esteemed surgeon I should say."

"Glad to make your acquaintance Doctor." There was a silent pause as the manager stood looking at the two customers. "Ah…How are your two dishes, gentlemen?"

"Excellent I should say. I don't know about the doctor's steak, looks burnt in my opinion."

"Well, let me take that back and have it done correctly, Doctor."

Slim put his hand over the steak. "It is just as I like it, Mr. Shagshaw."

"Jack, please. Okay," he said rubbing his hands together with mild excitement. "Then both of you are happy?"

"We are," the Governor said with a twist of his head.

"Thank you, gentlemen. I will leave you to your meal." Shagshaw turned and moved away.

The two ate in silence. Slim said nothing but scowled and shook his head. "Okay, okay…what's the punchline here? Billie Sampson, what about him?"

The Governor took another bite of his bass and then of the vegetables. He chewed deliberately looking across the table at the man. When he finished, he wiped his mouth with his cloth napkin, took another sip of the martini, and smiled at the man.

"Sampson is at UTMB as we speak. Turns out that he has just the right kidney courtesy of James "Slim" McCormack. Now when he has a stone, he goes into kidney failure and seizures and such. There were two lawyers in my office not a week ago. In addition to ridiculous calls for clemency, they claim malpractice on your part, that is taking the left kidney out when active stones were still in the right. Now they are upset, and why they would represent such a reprehensible piece of humanity is something I will never understand. But represent they do, jurisprudence being what it is."

"I don't understand why you're involved, Von?"

"Yes, I don't either, but these two lawyers are persistent, and they made their way into my office. They have a case, I am sorry to say. My advisors say malpractice for the plaintiff is a slam dunk. The damages they are throwing around. Woo…Weee, James can you imagine 10 million dollars, to a death row inmate? What kind of political hit does the state take for that, and me as well?"

Slim pushed his half-eaten plate across the table. "This is nonsense. I did what I thought was right. He never passed right sided stones according to him."

"Do you have that documented?"

"Well, not really but it is the truth."

"Well, he passes right sided kidney stones now and quite often."

"What do you want me to do, Von?"

The Governor finished his bass. He took a large drink from his martini. "I think you are going to need to retire James, maybe disappear. They can still go after you, but we can control the award."

"Retire! You must be kidding! Let them sue. I have malpractice insurance for these sort of issues."

"Issues, do you know what type of exposure I am facing here. I am the Governor whose brother is an incompetent fool. You know this is not your first foray into malpractice here."

And with that, it was on the table. Years back Slim had been cited for drunkenness in public. That led to a trumped-up malpractice suit by a disgruntled patient, settled in the plaintiff's favor. It was a fact, though, one well-documented in the public record. In reality, another lawsuit would ruin him, insurance or not. One surrounded by such high-powered people would be a disaster.

Slim hung his head. He knew what the Governor was saying was right. "I'll need to think about this, speak to Lucille, Von. I have a family to support."

The Governor handed Slim a business card. "This lawyer is a tough dog. He will advise you and work out the best benefits and settlement. His fee will be fed to me, I will take care of it." The Governor wiped his mouth with his napkin. He stood for a moment and looked down on Slim. He then signaled to his assistant and walked out of the restaurant.

As he passed, Shagshaw nodded and tried to greet the man on his way out. The manager had a questioning expression on his face as the Governor exited. He looked across the restaurant at Slim. He reached for a business card that was pinned to the wall and dialed the phone.

"Jennifer Harry please. Yes, are you Jennifer Harry of KTRK?"

Chapter 15

Jennifer Harry put the receiver down after speaking to Jack Shagshaw. The call was just what she was looking for. Reviewing her handwritten notes, she flipped back in the spiral notebook and studied.

First, where did Harry recall the name? She grabbed a manila file off her crowded desk and flipped through cut out news articles.

"Yes, there is the name, Sara Jean Shagshaw, Sampson's victim." The two, the manager Jack Shagshaw and the victim, shared the same last name. Jennifer would have to research the connection. She moved to the microfiche machine and scanned back on newspaper articles from the time of the murder. Sure enough in the caption to a funeral picture a mourning Jack Shagshaw was mentioned as the father of the deceased.

Next, she wondered how the man got her phone number? He said he had her card, and she remembered distantly giving it to a man at the funeral. Shagshaw mentioned being the owner of Shagshaw's Steak Restaurant. He just served the state's Governor and overheard a conversation with Slim McCormack. Here retirement and malpractice concerning Billie Sampson were discussed. McCormack was not happy. This was a big story. She picked up her things and moved to speak to her manager.

"Scott, I just got off of the phone with Jack Shagshaw, the father of the murdered Sara Jean Shagshaw."

"So," the man said. Scott was a little balding man, with small wireless rim glasses perched on his nose. He was always drinking a Styrofoam cup of old coffee. Scott was an adequate journalist, but difficult to work with. He was sitting at a small gun-metal gray desk loaded with piles and piles of paperwork.

"He overheard a conversation with Von W. Mitchel, the Governor, and doctor James McCormack. He heard the word malpractice and retirement, Scott!"

"Who is he? And whose retirement?"

"He is Shagshaw. The Governor was talking about a large malpractice settlement concerning McCormack's surgery on Billie James Sampson, the death row murderer. The doctor removed Sampson's left kidney leaving him with real trouble with the right. It's come to the point of requiring an enormous reconstructive surgery for the man at UTMB. The source indicates that the Governor insisted on Slim's retirement. I have heard that Felix Artain and Luther Johnson are representing the inmate and have been in the Governor's office. So the suit makes sense.

"See what confirmation you can get here. Talk to the lawyers. Contact Mitchel's office for approval, though they likely will drag their feet."

Felix Artain's office was across town in a baby blue and white restored Victorian building. Jennifer Harry parked her rusted VW bug along the curb, grabbed her leopard colored backpack and entered the office.

"May I help you," a beautiful young receptionist asked the reporter.

"Here is my card, is Mr. Artain in?"

The receptionist studied the card carefully. She pushed a button and picked up the receiver. "Mr. Artain, a Jennifer Harry from KTRK is here and wishes to speak to you. Okay." Holding the phone to her chest, she asked. "What brings you to see Mr. Artain?"

"Billie James Sampson," was the single phrase answer.

The woman relayed the name to the lawyer. "He will see you, just enter through this door," the receptionist led Jennifer through two heavy doors and into the office.

"Mr. Artain, I understand you represent Billie James Sampson." Harry shook the man's hand and took a seat in front of his desk.

"I don't have a lot of time, Ms. is it Harry?"

"Yes, I'll get to the point then." Harry pulled out her ringed notebook and a pencil. "What can you tell me about Billie James Sampson?"

"We, my partner and I represent him. What exactly are you inquiring about?"

"Rumor is that the removal of his left kidney by James McCormack is being litigated, a malpractice suit. Can you confirm that?"

"Well, that is a matter of public record so yes, we are arguing that the removal of his kidney was below the standard of care and resulted in predictable complications. We filed papers just this week."

"And the plaintiff is doctor James McCormack?"

"Yes, he is. He should be served soon."

"Damages, what are the damages you are requesting."

"Well, one million dollars. And by the way, we are citing the Governor in this litigation.

"How is the Governor libel?"

"Read the complaint. Now I must excuse myself." Artain stood and ushered the reporter out of his office.

☞

"I'll have the meatloaf." The elderly woman with thick black glasses and hair pulled back in a black hairnet, served the white-coated man without a smile. "Thank you." He took his tray and stood quietly in the line waiting to pay.

"James McCormack?" A man in a black suit with a clip-on dark tie tapped him on the shoulder and questioned?

"Yes. Do I know you?"

"Then these are for you," said the man as he shoved a thick wad of papers in a manila envelope onto McCormack's tray, landing in the mashed potatoes. He then turned and walked away.

McCormack looked at the envelope with grief. He wiped it with his white coat and placed it into the right pocket. The cafeteria patrons before and behind him smiled an uncomfortable smile, each customer returning his stare with embarrassment. The surgeon expected it, however, a thick packet of thanks from the local court. It was a delivery one wished would disappear, along with himself. Without opening it, the man was confident of the contents.

McCormack paid for his meal after waiting patiently in line, moved to an overfull trash can and ceremoniously dumped his uneaten food tray. A boy stood by the canister and examined the discarded dish with a question on his brow. "Hey, mister?" Was heard as McCormack left. He exited the cafeteria, rode the elevator to the fourth floor, and entered his office in silence.

James "Slim" McCormack's life was unraveling rapidly, even before he was processed served. This, unfortunately, was not the only service of late. A plaintiff-successful malpractice suit two years before. Divorce was ongoing in a nasty dirt filled proceeding. His only daughter, Fiona, was caught up in a drug-infested life. His alcoholism was overcoming him, drinking day and night. However, it was his medical practice that was wallowing away his life. Overworked, over-burdened, underappreciated, and for the first time, he did not value his life's chosen profession. Medicine was a noble profession. It was a principled vocation, one of worthiness; a decent and upright career. For the first time, he did not feel that way.

The hours were long, the pressures overwhelming at times. McCormack's confidence was in tatters. One wrong move in the operating room and hell was to pay. His surgeon's life had come just to this, a job, and never could just a job repay him for his feelings of late.

He stood in the dark office and looked at his framed diploma hanging on the wall. In the glass was his shadowy reflections, a pitiful excuse for a physician as well as a man, he thought.

He read its inscription. *The University of Texas Medical Branch at Galveston confirms Doctor of Medicine on James Simpson McCormack.* Anger billowed up. He struck the glass frame with his balled fist, cracked glass, and a bloody knuckle the result.

He dropped into his desk chair and put his head on his desk. McCormack panted in panic, closing his eyes and hoping to fall quickly asleep. Without success, he lifted his head and reached into the lower left drawer. Drawing out a half-finished bottle of Jack Daniels, he poured a full glass and downed it with three deep swallows.

Remembering the manila envelope, he pulled it from his white coat. He read the contents rapidly confirming that this was a malpractice suit for his surgical removal of Billie James Sampson's left kidney with ten million dollars cited in damages. In the end, however, he was thrown for another setback. In a section entitled Dereliction of Duty one Von William Mitchel was specified. Allegations of Gross Negligence, Recklessness, Breached duty of reasonable care, know or should have known that one James Simpson McCormack, brother in blood, was negligent for years with a regular practice of alcohol-related malpractice.

It was as if he was hit in the gut. He never imagined that his half-brother Von would be cited in this legal complaint. This magnified the complexity and assured a feeding frenzy with the media.

He replaced the papers in the manila envelope and returned it to his coat pocket. He was panicking again. Cold sweat covered his brow, a sick feeling in the pit of his stomach. His mouth was so dry that his tongue stuck to the roof of his palate.

McCormack reached to his keys and unlocked the right lower drawer of his desk. He removed a wooden box which he set before him. Within was a 357 Smith and Wesson handgun. He checked that the chambers which were full. He cried replacing his head on the desk. McCormack inserted the barrel of the gun in his mouth and fired a single shot into the roof of his mouth exiting through the back of his skull.

Chapter 16

White-coated beings stood silently at the foot of his bed staring at the patient. It was dawn, still, and dark in the room; the only light coming from the hallway lights which back-lit the group as an angelic assembly.

The patient awoke hours before, cowering under the sheet, spooked, and afraid of the man in black. It was several hours since that demon appeared, tormenting, laughing and jumping to his anguish. The beast touched him hideously, shaking and bringing the angry response of chest compressions and vicious alchemy. Then he would sit snickering and smug on his perch above the room, red mascara eyes, long white hands with sharp twisted nails. He spat out vile words and coughed revolting phlegm. But then he was gone, at least it seemed an episode of malicious malevolence, calmed for the time being.

"Mr. Sampson," Dana said standing in the center of the well-scrubbed group. She appeared tense, her hands balled into fists within her white coat pockets. "How is the patient this morning," she said with expectation in her voice.

The patient, Billie James Sampson, pulled the white sheet to his chin in defense. He stared at the woman in silence, fear in his light blue eyes.

"What about his vital signs Mark?"

Intern Mark Upham grabbed the bedside chart. "He's afebrile with stable BP pulse and respirations over 24 hours." Here he reported the absence of fever, with blood pressure, pulse, and respiration all stable over the last day.

Dana stepped forward slowly with deliberation. She looked to the group for encouragement as she did so. Dana carefully took the sheet from the man's hands and pulled it down revealing his eagle tattooed chest. She took her red stethoscope from her pocket. Ironically, it was capped with a tiny stuffed bear, loved by pediatric patients. Dana listened to the man's lungs, heart, and abdomen. Inspecting the mid-line wound, she found it healing well and intact.

She began to kneel down and look at the urine Foley bag on the floor but stopped herself. She checked the leather restraints on Sampson's arms and then cautiously continued. The urine was cloudy with mucous. Dana picked up the bag and showed it to the group. "The urine has pieces of mucous in it. Anyone know why?"

An eager medical student piped up. "He has had an ileal ureter, where ileum bowel replaces the ureter. The mucous is from that loop of bowel."

"Correct," Dana said. She smiled at the group, someone had been listening. She stood and looked at the patient, then moved back to the foot of the bed.

"Have you passed any gas, Mr. Sampson?"

"Thhhhhhhhhhhhh," a huge flatus vibrated out from the man seeming to lift the covers. A foul smell slowly pervaded the small room. "Like that Doctor Rausch?" A friendly smile slowly crossed Sampson's frightened face. The event seemed to relax the man. He acknowledged the group as if he knew they were advocates for his care.

Quiet laughs around the group reinforced the appropriateness of the process. "The patient has flatus," was repeated by the assembly. After abdominal surgery, the bowel goes to sleep so to speak, a process called ileus. The presence of flatus indicates that the gut is functioning again.

Dana moved again to Sampson's bedside. She gently pulled the sheet up around his neck covering him completely. Sampson placed his leather bound hand on hers. Dana pulled back at first with concern. She looked at the man, deep into his eyes and replaced her hand with his.

Turning to Mark, she asked about the man's cardiac enzymes drawn yesterday in response to the apparent cardiac event. Cardiac enzymes are sensitive measurements of heart injury. Given the episode of arrhythmia and the trauma from CPR these would be expected to be elevated. " All of them were normal somehow, Dana."

Dana moved back to the group and looked at Mark's clipboard. "How could that be, he had a run of V-fib, a distinct cardiac arrest and a long bout of CPR?".

"I don't know, but they were normal."

"Okay to start his diet, clear liquids?" Dana said to Lee W. who shook his head affirmatively. "Mr. Sampson we are starting you on food, just liquids at first!"

Sampson pulled himself up on the bed. He was thrilled, and a broad-faced smile showed so. Soon, however, he was cowering again, sheet pulled up under his chin with two hands gripping the white cloth tensely. "What about the man?"

Dana looked at each of the group. "What man, Mr. Sampson?"

Sampson shook his head. He appeared worried that the man in black would return. He was terrified of the being, and feared what he might represent, death.

"The man in black." Sampson sat up starkly in bed and looked around the room for the demon-man with fright on his face. "He split," he said relieved as he lay down again gingerly.

"Must be talking about one of the guards, I guess." Dana thought to herself about this man in black. Given the normal cardiac enzymes, she wondered whether the event was supernatural.

The group turned and began to leave the room.

"Doctor Rausch, I needs to talk at you?"

Dana hung back. Again with reluctance, she moved to the bedside. She looked to the group which was exiting the room. "Go ahead I'm okay." Alongside the man, she focused on his leather restraints.

"I knows you afraid of me! Right on Doc, I hear you. I's so wrong. Can't you be okay with me again?" Sincerity was apparent. The man really wanted the Doctor to forgive his attempted rape. The demon-man had gotten him. Death was the being's wish, and he had induced the cardiac event to torment Sampson. Plague the man he did, leading to CPR, a frightening occurrence where he was totally out of control.

Dana looked down at the floor. She seemed to review the events of the last weeks. She reached to her neck and fingered the scar left during her assault.

Dana looked at the man controlled with leather restraints. She appeared to think about Sampson. He was really pitiful. A death row inmate convicted of felony assault and brutally beating a young girl to her death. But, it was her nature to forgive, and she found herself doing so. She shook her head affirmatively and placed her hand in his big hand.

"I feel safe with the leather restraints, Mr. Sampson. Will you not touch me like that again?"

Tears came to Sampson. He looked up at Dana and shook his head affirmatively. All the bravado was gone, a broken man now a threat to no one.

༺༻

The funeral happened on a cold rainy day in Conroe Texas. It was wet, stormy, and poorly attended. A memorial service preceded the committal at the gravesite. Here the rain pelted down on the attendees, curved black tarred streets winding between tall trees and ancient white cement grave markers.

Several law related issues ended that day. Lucille McCormack, the decedent's wife, was the sole member of the dead man's family to attend, a bitter divorce in the process now not necessary. The daughter was hospitalized after a heroin overdose. Her addiction was quite profound, her father's suicide pushing her over the edge. Slim's portion of the malpractice suit was satisfied that day. With his death, there was no primary defendant. It was not completely settled, however, the Governor's responsibility awaiting procedural issues with the plaintiff's lawyers.

The small family gathering at the burial site began, only to be interrupted by the Governor's motorcade. The small group turned to see a black limousine arrive and Texas Rangers surrounding the Governor's vehicle. He stood by the limo and did not interact with the service.

Debra Harry attended that afternoon. When she saw the Governor, she moved to his side.

"Governor, I am Debra Harry of KTRK. Can I ask you about the status of the Dereliction of Duty portion of James McCormack's Malpractice Suit? "

"No, you cannot. Harry, it's my brother's funeral Gxx Dxxx it?"

With that, the Governor slipped into the limousine and drove off, and the committal continued.

Chapter 17

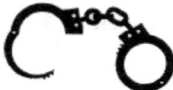

Billie James Sampson shuffled slowly down the TDCJ's hallway. He was assisted by a nurse, a manacled man aided by a smallish woman dressed in white. He was a tall, thin muscular man, dressed in blah-colored mustard pajamas. On his feet were two hospital-issued black cut pile, loose-fitting slippers, worn over white cotton socks. Gun-toting correctional officers eyed him carefully as they walked on each side of the shackled man.

"Three times a day Billie, each time walking farther down the hall," the nurse said encouraging him.

"But it hurts it does." He pointed to his abdomen with the thumb of his secured hand as he hobbled along.

"Well, you're due for a pain shot after your walk."

The man smiled a golden tine smile as he said: "Give me some Morph, Sally."

The group finished in the man's room, one officer standing by the door while the other assisted him into bed. Sampson was a death-row inmate, one whose security was critical. The attempted rape during his hospital stay was a black mark on the TDCJ. So the officers were unusually careful with the man. As per protocol, they uncuffed him, first his legs, allowing him to swing into bed, followed by his hands. The chain around his midriff was then unlocked and removed.

Lee W. Hickok watched from the TDCJ's nursing station. He was waiting for the man, who fascinated him, the evil now superimposed over an apparent revelation. He was interested in talking to him in some detail, and so he took this Wednesday, his educational half-day to do so.

Standing in the doorway, he looked at Sampson. The nurse was finishing up with him, giving an intramuscular injection of pain medicine.

"Mr. Sampson, its doctor Hickok," Lee W. said, walking to the foot of the bed.

"Oh…Hi, doc. Just got my morph."

Lee W. pulled a chair to his bedside and sat looking at the man. Billie had changed. No longer was he angry and intimidating. "How are you, that is after surgery?"

"Doing okay. Got liquids for breakfast. I's hungry for something real, though."

"Soon. Did you tolerate the liquids okay?"

"I's downed it all doc. Salty."

"You'll be out of here in no time Mr. Sampson." With that, Lee W. caught himself. Would this man ever be *out of here?* He remembered his history and date with the needle and wished he hadn't said that.

Sampson grimaced. He looked at the ground beside him and said nothing.

"Sorry, Well I mean going back to the Walls." Lee W. sat up straight in the chair.

Sampson looked up and shook his head affirmatively.

"Billie, can I call you Billie?"

"That's my name, doc."

"Billie, you mentioned a man in black when we rounded, what did you mean by that?"

Fear came over Billie's face. He quickly washed that look away and met Lee W.'s stare.

"Oh, I am sorry, but could you tell me something about that experience?"

"Real bad, doc." Billie hung his head. He nervously rubbed his closely cropped head. "Ya, that's a real bad dude." He thought for a moment. "See, he was all in black. Had these red eyes and these long twisted sharp nails. Sitting right up there for the longest time and laughing at me, he was." He pointed to the corner of the room, and the wall mounted television.

Lee W. was gripped by the thought. "Who was he, Billie?"

There was silence for a moment as the man thought about a miserable time. "I's don't know. Best I know, the Devil. You know, he would torture me. He would. I ain't lying. He injected me with heart-stopping stuff, doc." Billie looked straight at Lee W. with a wisp of fear in his face.

This was something new, and Lee W.'s interest was wetted. "Before your heart arrest, he injected you?"

"Ya Sir. I swear he puts something in my IV and next thing I know they're pounding on my chest. It hurts real bad it does, doc. Them pushing and pounding all over me."

Lee W. paused and thought. He wasn't especially averse to the existence of demons, but the thought of one here in the hospital was somewhat odd. "Well, I am sorry Billie. It is evident that this Devil tormented you. Did it scare you?"

Billie laughed very quietly, shook his head slowly and said nothing.

"Now you said nails. You mean he had long fingernails?"

"Ya…and he keeps waving his hands and laughing at me. And black hair, you know long and real dirty like."

There was silence in the room as the two thought about the notion. "Well, that must have been terrible. What did you learn, yaw-all seem different, Billie."

The man smiled, sort of proud of himself. "Ya, I's different Doc. Those things I's did. Doc I was real bad! Now I's just want to live, but I's going to die soon. Sure wish the lady would like me."

"Billie, doctor Rausch says you asked her to be friends again."

With that, the man sat up and smiled. "Ya, the lady. I wrongs her for sure. Don't know why I did it." He dropped his head. "She is just…well…hot, you know. And me I'm stuck in here. Just did it. But I's real wrong. Do you think she can like me again?"

"She's an amazing woman. I think if you behave she will forgive you."

Billie sat back in his bed a huge smile on his face. "Wow, if I was out of here, with her, but I know I's got to behave."

Billie looked as if he was going to say something for the longest time. "I know I ain't long for this world." He looked down at the floor. "I know they's going give me the needle, and soon. It will be before I know it. Doc, I's got no friends in the world. No family. Mom, she's gone, my old man, he's gone and I better for it. I ain't married. Got no old lady anymore. Everyone left me. And I don't blame them, I don't. What I's saying…it's hard, but would you attend?"

"Attend?" Lee W. thought long and hard. "You mean the execution don't you?"

He reached into a box of tissue on his nightstand and blew his nose, then looked Lee W. in the eyes. "Ya. I hate's to ask. You know you so *portant*, but I got no one doc!"

"I would be honored, Billie." Lee W. stood and grabbed the man's hand for a handshake. As he left the room, he eyed the television in the upper corner of the room. He could have sworn that the frame was drooping like something heavy had sat on it. He stopped at the nursing station and ordered Billie a regular diet.

Chapter 18

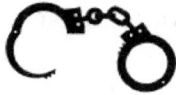

"Well then give him a sleeper Sally. How's chloral hydrate 500 milligrams."

"He doesn't want one. It's like he is afraid of going to sleep, doctor Upham. You know the way he gets."

"Should I come see him then? I am really busy, but maybe it would help."

Mark Upham, MD was the intern for the urology service and on call. Each night since Billie James Sampson's surgery, the patient refused to go to sleep. Upham had gotten in the habit of visiting the man before bed, in part because he could visit Sally, but tonight he was so busy. The operating room was going, doctors Hickok and Dana Rausch exploring a gunshot wound to the kidney. Then there were admission history and physicals, all kind of scut work, and the emergency room would not leave him alone. He felt he should try, though, swing by and help the man go to sleep.

The TDCJ was closed at that time, and the strict correctional officers would not allow him in. Upham, however, knew a back way into the fortress. Through the cafeteria, up the back elevator, outside for a moment, then up the stairs to the eighth floor. It was a walk typical of an intern's life.

Sampson was in bed when Upham arrived. The patient was a frightening bundle of contradictions. Extreme violence on the one hand, but sadness underneath. Upham had grown to like the man. The story of his brutal beating of a woman in a bar parking lot was hard to condone. And then the assault of doctor Rausch, he remembered that day. She made the mistake of visiting the man on her own. He remembered seeing her afterward. Disheveled and emotionally distraught, the event rocketed around the medical center. Rausch took the occurrence with such strength, never even copping out on rounding on the man. She acted as if it never happened, and never reneged on her responsibilities.

Sampson was a different man now, however. The man definitely changed. Rumor was that he saw a demon during his cardiac arrest. If you could sense fear by looking at a person, then it just might be true.

He was sitting in his bed with the head raised, all the lights in the room on, his radio turned up listening to the Hoston Astros. Upham stood in the doorway and observed the man.

"Time for bed Mr. Sampson."

"Not just yet, dude." Sampson looked relieved when the intern announced himself. "I's just afraid to go to sleep you know?

"What keeps you awake?"

"The man in black, he comes back."

Upham decided to try and get into this phenomenon. "What did this guy look like?"

Sampson was frightened even talking about the demon. He was silent for the longest time.

"Black, evil, greasy, and he hates me. Ya, he does. Sat right up there on the TV and laughed at me."

"Was he real?"

"Real as anything I's seen before. Had red eyes like dripping, and long twisted fingers." Sampson said wringing his hands.

Sally arrived with Sampson's sleeper. "Will you take the sleeping pill, Mr. Sampson?

"I's don't know. The man might come back in my dream." Fright was evident on the rough man's face.

"It's critical to get sleep, especially when your healing from surgery." Upham sat forward in his chair and adamantly tried to convince the man.

"Okay's I's take it. You stay till I's asleep doctor Upham?"

Sally handed the medicine cup with the chloral hydrate to Sampson. Upham shook his head yes. Sampson downed the drug. Within minutes the man was asleep.

A smudged purple horizon framed a setting red sun and confronted the man, as he stumbled along a twisted desert path marked by scrub brush and black dalea. Red-tailed Hawks flew a menacing flight overhead, with caws of predatory supremacy. A hot breeze blew confrontation forward, it was scorching, and he was parched with thirst. A hawk attempted to land on his shoulder, a frightening attack that he violently brushed away.

He appeared beside him suddenly, a demon dressed in a black Victorian turn of the century outfit with knee height black shiny boots and a wooden maple cane. A cake white pasty complexion outlined his hideous face. Red dripping mascara plotted the eyes, long sharp eye-teeth punctuated a sick expression of hate.

His hands defined the demon, always in motion looking for a site to land. They were covered with white skin, blue radiating veins and twisted long pointing nails. The demon continuously brushed back his greasy black hair and straightened imaginary wrinkles in his garments.

The demon placed a hand on the shoulder of the man. Like opposite battery poles, the man rejected his touch as if a negative field of force.

"Who the Hell are you?"

"Hahahaha....," was the demon's long hideous reply. "I am you, have you not figured that out yet? And by the way, Hell's the proper word."

The man stood staring at his repulsive self. It fit, he realized, gawking, he was looking at some kind of mirror-image. A being of his deeper self; filthy, disgusting, and hideous but somehow himself. The demon violently grabbed his neck with the curved end of his cane and tossed him to the ground with a start, his face now reflecting an image in the monster's black boots.

He tried to lift himself, held by the cane, pounded and milled down by the man's sharp-nailed hand. But he could not rise. Instead, he was forced to concentrate on his image in the boots.

He soon realized that he was looking into his facial image. Eyes: light blue irises surrounded by the red mascara. His teeth: shiny nearly golden sharp. The image nauseated him, and he vomited on the ground. The demon released the pressure from the cane, and the man stood slowly and backed away.

He raced away down the twisted path. He looked behind, his adversary calmly disappearing. As he moved along, he shook, hurrying away and separating himself.

The reverie continued, however, heat blowing him along the warped path. The sky darkened, and fire rose from the ground in front of him. Before him was the discarded baseball bat, wooden and fierce, still with pieces of brain attached to its worn surface.

Chapter 19

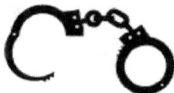

When he awoke, everything was wonderfully different. The room, the overhead music; all that he loathed, even his captors were suddenly okay. The sun's earliest rays leaked through the window blind like a wonderful aura, and he noticed for the first time in forever that he was happy. Tears dripped down his toughened face. He wiped them quickly to avoid detection, almost embarrassed at their presence. His childhood came to mind. In the past it was always foddering for self-hate; the memories of his crowded beat down rat-trap home returned. He remembered the dirty smell of urine and the mindless crack of the television across the room where his drunken beast of a father was passed out and snoring. The man beat and raped him for pleasure until he grew to return the favor. Now, after years of hatred, it no longer seemed relevant to the hardened man.

He took a deep breath in his new life. Blistering pain in the abdominal incision resulted, but even that was tolerable. With difficulty he sat up on the bed, his legs bound with chains.

"Hey boss, I's got's to pee."

"Ya, Sampson I'll get to you." After some time, the officer entered the room. He locked Sampson's wrists to his waist, and slowly unlocked his leggings. The prisoner struggled to his feet, moved to the doorless restroom and voided.

"Pus, there's pus in my pee, boss," Sampson said as he returned to his bed.

"I don't care if there are razors in your piss Sampson!" The officer locked his bindings, tightening them up with a smile.

"Books, I have books for your pleasure Mr. Sampson!" The elderly woman with a limp and a pushcart full of books was here again at his door. She was a plumpish elderly woman, dressed in a red striped dress with medical grade nylon stockings and curly greying hair. To her, books were a treasure, her smile, and love for them visible. Sampson had never thought about her, but today was different.

"Ya gots something for a slow reader?" The truth was that the man could not read, he had trouble enough speaking. To read, however, that was suddenly something that he wanted to do with all his heart.

Both officers stood and gently restrained the woman from entering. "Ma'am you can't go into that room."

The woman looked up at them and smiled. "Heavens why not? He wants to read, gentlemen!"

The lead officer looked at his subordinate. With a head signal to stay at the door, he moved to the bedside. After checking the man's wrist cuffs, he moved a chair for the woman and beckoned for her to join him.

The woman limped into the room pushing her heavy cart. She stood and perused her stock, selecting a book. She opened the volume and read some text.

We went tiptoeing along a path amongst the trees back towards
the end of the widow's garden, stooping down so as the branches
wouldn't scrape our heads.

She then handed the book to the man. Sampson opened it to the title page. For the longest time, he stared at the writing. "The...ad...of...Huck...ber...Finn?"

The woman stood and moved to his side. She pointed to the title. *"The Adventures of Huckleberry Finn.* You would love it but maybe later Mr. Sampson." She turned to her cart. In the corner was a thin illustrated book which she handed to the man.

A smile appeared on his face as he held the text, looking at its cover. *"The Cat in the Hat?"* He looked up at the woman and laughed. "I's seen this before!"

"Well, Mr. Sampson you could start with this. It is very entertaining!"

And so the hardened criminal, a murderer, and rapist began:

"The sun did not shine. it was too wet to play. So we sat in the house all that cold, cold, wet day."

"That brings us to Billie James Sampson. Mark, can you present him?" Tuesday and Thursday department rounds consisted of the presentation of all patients on the urologic service at UTMB in the departmental library. At the meeting, this morning, was Lee W., Dana Rausch, Duke McHugh, Mark Upham, various attending from the department, and the medical students on the service.

"Ya, well Sampson is a 23-year-old black male who is three days status post ileal ureter. He is in post-op day number seven. A cardiac arrest on post-op day number one occurred, but resuscitation was successful. Since this episode, he has been doing well. His vital signs are stable, he is afebrile, and now he is on a regular diet. He has a right nephrostomy tube, and this is the right nephrostogram done this morning with antibiotic coverage." Upham placed the images up on an x-ray box for the group to review. These showed images of dye entering the right kidney nephrostomy tube, with x-rays taken to view the ileal loop of bowel functioning as his right ureter.

Dana stood and moved to the view box, pulling a telescopic pointer out of her coat. "You see the contrast moving out of the nephrostomy tube and filling the ileal loop. Later films show that the loop is well filled and the contrast fills the bladder promptly. Post-drainage films show no extravasation."

Dana described the x-ray study for the group. The nephrostomy tube and the ileal ureter were functioning well.

"We will clamp the nephrostomy tube tomorrow and take it out in a day or so if he does well."

Upham went on to the next patient.

"Let's run over to TDCJ and see Sampson, Dana." Lee W. asked Dana after the conference, and the two journeyed over to the prison ward. The sky was a beautiful blue, with a light sea breeze as they made their way across the bridge to TDCJ. There ID's were checked, and the two entered the facility making their way to Sampson's room.

What they saw amazed them, and they stood in the doorway watching the prisoner and his guest.

> *I sat there with sally.*
> *we sat there, we two.*
> *and i said, 'how i wish*
> *we had something to do!'*

"Now you read Mr. Sampson."

> "I's sat th…ere with sally,
> We sat th…ere, we two,
> And I said, 'how I wish
> We had some…thin to do!"

The woman with the limp sat at Sampson's bedside holding *The Cat in the Hat,* patiently correcting the prisoner man.

"Now don't say I's, there is not an s, it is just I sat. Say there all in one word you know that word. And it is thing not thin."

Sampson sat in bed. His wrists were shackled. He had a pair of thick black reading glasses on and was holding a thin brightly colored book in his right hand. He looked up at the two physicians, with a confident smile on his face. He returned his concentration to the woman, looking at her name badge.

"Carol, is your name Carol?"

"Why yes, read it all. Carol Winegarten."

"Carol Wine…garden?"

"Winegarten."

"Glad to meet ya, Carol Winegarten. Billie Sampson." Sampson lifted his shackled hand in an encumbered wave. He looked up from the book at the two physicians standing in the door. A big sincere smile came over his face. "Dr. Hickok and Dr. Rausch, how are you this fine day?" He looked intently at Dana, a wondering look on his face.

Lee W. turned to Dana with a curious smile. The two entered the room, moving to the patient's bedside. Carol smiled and said: "I have a real learner here Dr. Hickok. Mr. Sampson is reading!"

"I don't want to interrupt," said Lee W. "Could we ask your student some questions?"

"Why certainly." Carol took the book, stood returning it to her cart. "We are about done here for the day. I will return tomorrow, Mr. Sampson."

Sampson smiled and thanked the woman. "You will really come here tomorrow?" He said with some concern.

"She looked at her watch. "Yes, I'll come earlier than today so as to not interfere with your Dr.'s." And with that, she left pushing her book cart out of the room.

Dana was all smiles. "You are reading Mr. Sampson?"

Sampson said nothing but smiled a happy smile. He shook his head affirmatively all the while looking at Dana.

She reached without thought to her scar on her neck and quickly returned her hand to her side. There was the usual element of fear on her face, but just for a moment as a large smile returned.

"That is wonderful. *The Cat in the Hat*, what a story! *Green Eggs and Ham* is my favorite Mr. Sampson."

There was silence in the room. Embarrassment crossed the prisoner's face. Sampson looked down and said nothing for a while. He looked up wondering about Dana. "Dr. Rausch, can I talk to you sometime?"

Dana looked at Lee W. searching for support in his face. Turning now and facing the man she said: "you can talk to me now, Mr. Sampson."

"Will ya'se call me Billie?" He looked down at his shackled hands.

"Okay, Billie, what do you need?" Dana wondered.

It was hard for the man to speak in full sentences. He was quite troubled by what he needed to say. "Ah…ah…I's so sorry Dr. Rausch for what I's done to you." He rubbed his hands on his thighs. "I…I…don't know why I would do that?"

Dana's face turned a bright red. She too looked down not knowing what to say. There were several seconds of silence in the room. "I don't know either, Billie!"

Sampson looked up. "I's was a different man, Dr. Rausch! I...I...I's was evil." He dropped his head. "I have no scuse, I did it to ya, and I never forgive myself."

Dana stood in silence. She really seemed to have nothing to say.

Finally, Sampson said: "I pray for you. I hope you'se alright."

Chapter 20

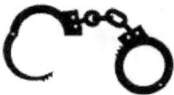

The letter arrived in the departmental mail one day in April. It was about eight years after Billie's discharge from UTMB, the return address reading just Huntsville Unit, 815 12th St, Huntsville, TX 77348.

In the interim JD, Dr. Wilson that is, kept me informed of his medical progress through periodic letters. At first, these summaries arrived every month or so and then eventually annually. They noted his condition, primarily urologic.

My impression was that he was doing well. The ileal ureter seemed to function as it was intended, keeping him from having episodes of kidney stone pain and obstructive failure of his solitary kidney. Life moves on, however, and I realized that I had not thought of the man in quite some time.

I sat at my desk, a pile of mail with Billie's letter on top. I pulled JD's last letter from my top drawer to review his case. Dated August 21, 1992, the letter read as follows:

Lee W, I examined Billie James Sampson last week and dictated the following:

BJS is a 36-year-old black male inmate.

History of present illness: Patient states that he is doing well medically. He occasionally feels some mild right flank discomfort after which he passes a small stone in his mucous stained urine. Otherwise, he is without complaints.

Past Medical History: Patient has solitary right kidney and medullary sponge kidney with a long complicated renal stone history.

Past Surgical History: Multiple stone associated surgeries including an ileal ureter replacement surgery at UTMB in 1985.

Family History: non-contributory

Physical Exam:

Height 6 foot 2 inches, Weight is stable at 203 pounds. Blood pressure is 124 over 73 mm of mercury, pulse 68, with respiration 16 per minute. He is a well-developed black male in no apparent distress.

    Head, eyes, ears nose and throat: normocephalic

    Chest: Clear to auscultation

    Cardiac: Heart rate and rhythm normal, no rubs or murmurs.

    Abdomen: Well healed midline abdominal incision. Normal bowel sounds. No masses or hepatosplenomegaly.

    Genitourinary: normal male external genitalia. Normal digital rectal exam, guaiac negative.

    Extremities: No cyanosis, clubbing, or edema.

    Impression: Male inmate in medically stable condition.

    Plan: Return to clinic in one year.

    JD Wilson, MD

I read the plan over and over again. RTC in one year. One year, in a death row inmate, I wondered how many he had left, especially with the letter arriving.

I sliced open the envelope and read what was a short note, printed in blue crayon.

    Dr. Hickok:

It will be soon now. I wonder if you could visit me some time like you said?

Sincerely,

Billie

I immediately picked up the phone and spoke to the librarian, Mrs. Hutchitt, and asked her to research the man. She returned my call the next day with this information. Billie James Sampson was scheduled to be executed, by lethal injection, the following Tuesday, just six days later.

It is crazy, I know, but I knew when I first received that letter, even before opening it, that I was going to see Billie. I told him, years before, that I would come. The execution, being scheduled for the next week, forced my decision. I spoke to Bill Ramport, the TDCJ director. He had connections at Huntsville and arranged a meeting with the inmate. I cleared my schedule, packed a bag and drove from Galveston in my 240 Z.

The city of Huntsville is 70 miles north of Houston and 170 miles south of Dallas. It sits within the Texas Triangle, the area of Texas outlined by the metropolitan areas of Austin, Dallas-Fort Worth and Houston. It is a city of 40,000, the Government seat of

Walker County Texas. It is up the I45 from Galveston; 120 miles, a two-hour drive. Mrs. Hutchitt put together an audio dossier on Sampson, which I listened to in my cassette tape deck on the way.

Billie James Sampson was born in Odessa Texas on May 5th, 1957 to two parents who did not want him. Lizzy Tolton died, soon after Billie's birth, she was a prostitute and succumbed to a drug overdose. His Father, Thomas Sampson raised him, so to speak. His male figure and head of the household was ruined by severe alcoholism. In addition, court documents accused him of repeatedly raping and beating Billie. However, one day Billie turned the tables and beat the man to near death with what would become his weapon of choice, a baseball bat.

Billie did not complete 9th grade but dropped out of High School at the age of 14 to begin a life of petty crime and violence. Court records place him in juvenile custody at the age of 15 for robbery and assault. His first felony was committed at the age of 20 and involved a violent sexual assault landing him a one-year stint in the Ector County Correctional Center in Odessa Texas. Years of run-ins with the law followed with internments in many of the fine Texas prison facilities.

On June 21, 1985, he raped and beat to death with his ball bat a young parent, Sara Jean Shagshaw at the Thirsty Thirties Beer and Pool dive in Lubbock Texas. The motive was not clear, he had met the girl before and elements of disrespect seemed likely. The court documents graphically depict her murder. She was lured into his car, where sex turned quickly to rape. Billie then beat her till she was unconscious. He tossed her out of the car, retrieved his bat from the trunk, and beat her beyond recognition. He drove away, crushing her wedding ring-laden hand with his rear tire.

Billie was picked up after a short investigation, tried in Lubbock County Civil Division, found guilty of first-degree murder and sentenced to death. Key to the investigation's case in support of first-degree murder was his baseball bat's presence in the locked trunk. He had planned the murder, the prosecution argued.

I listened to the librarian's dossier nearly the entire trip. She had included court pictures of the victim. An autopsy picture was particularly disturbing. In it, you could see her face. She was quite pretty, with blond long hair, but her skull was completely collapsed on the left side. In addition, there was a picture of her hand and innocent ringed finger after Billie's disrespectful exit from the scene. The violence was overwhelming.

I knew that Billie was a murderer but was unfamiliar with the violence of the case. I recalled his behavior in the hospital. I had a good window into his vicious personality. He actually demonstrated that violence, brutally assaulting Dana. I could not match that with my last image of the man, reading the Cat in the Hat with Carol Winegarten.

The death penalty is for me a complicated issue. Proponents of the death penalty say it is an important tool for preserving law and order, deters crime, and costs less than life imprisonment. They argue that retribution or "an eye for an eye" honors the victim, helps console grieving families, and ensures that the perpetrators of heinous crimes never have an opportunity to cause future tragedy.

Opponents of capital punishment, on the other hand, say it has no deterrent effect on crime, wrongly gives governments the power to take human life, and perpetuates social injustices by disproportionately targeting minorities and people who cannot afford good attorneys. They say lifetime jail sentences are a more severe and less expensive punishment than death.

Texans, in general, support the death penalty. I have mixed feelings, but primarily feel as the majority do. The main issue that bothers me is that there is a chance that an innocent man or woman could be executed. With modern DNA typing, however, this should not happen.

No matter the pros and cons, Billie James Sampson was going to be executed. My feelings seemed different that day as I knew, if you will, the *victim*.

Huntsville sits astride the I45 corridor. The prison, known as the walls unit because of its old brick façade, is at the south-east end of the town. I took the exit and quickly found myself in the prison facility. Driving down the access road I could already see signs of protest, positive and negative along the side of the road. "You must not execute God's child!" "Burn the criminal." And other similar signs lined the street.

I parked and registered with the TDCJ. Turned out that they were expecting a visit from me. Billie had prepared them. Day one was spent filling out bureaucratic forms, I would have to wait to the following day to see the inmate.

I checked into the Econo Lodge. At $53 per night, here was a bastion of heaven. It had a pool, a bed, and a shower and so I felt it met my needs. I had a greasy meal at the Happy Spoon and returned to my room for a swim. I had a feeling that sleep would be difficult that night.

Chapter 21

Lately, I have stopped praying. I still believe in its power, however. The magnitude of my task is haunting me, as I wait to see this man. And so, this night I return to the practice. My prayers are simple. I ask God to help me give some comfort to this man who is to be executed. For some reason, Billie James Sampson wants me present during this last period of his life. I could not tell you why at this point, but he did. Perhaps I could help him. I am doubtful. In my mind, I questioned whether I could help anyone through such an eventful episode.

In the past, my life was a certified mess. I am an alcoholic, a former 24/7 drinker. I am now 12 years sober. I have operated drunk so many times that for a while surgery was impossible, without being so. When I quit drinking, I self-treated my DT's with IV fluids and drugs. I was divorced but thankfully remarried to the same woman, Amber. My infidelities were frequent and with consequences. Her forgiveness is a miracle. I have one daughter, a 26-year-old named Kellie. She alternates between love for her dad and distaste.

Sleeping was tough that night as it often is when I am traveling. It was predictable, however, the dream etched in my psyche. It happened again, the recurrent dream that has haunted most of my life.

It is always the same. It is late at night. The moon lights my room in a frightening fashion through a torn window curtain. I am sleeping in my tiny bed when screaming and yelling wake me. I am very frightened. I get out of bed with my teddy bear friend, Boo. I go to my bedroom door and open it, reaching up above my head for the doorknob. The hallway is dark and cold, and the yelling becomes louder. I follow down the hallway, in search of the noise. Generally, I find my parents who are violently fighting. This night my dad is beating my Mother with his belt. She runs outside, grabs me and Boo, and takes us outside to our car. A chase ensues. True to the sad events of my childhood, my Father crashes into us and kills my Mother while I watch her die, her blood spattered on my face.

This night the dream is different. I wander down the hallway to a room without an exit, with no windows, and no door. It has shiny white walls, constructed of square polished tile. It is cold inside, there is a medicinal smell to the room. I am now dressed in a white surgical scrub suit.

In my hand is a large scalpel handle with a huge 22 blade. It is for protection, it is obvious to me, not for surgical work but protection.

In the corner is a large clapboard, stained wooden chair. There is someone sitting in that chair with their back towards me. The person is struggling, straps surrounding his head and trunk. The yelling has stopped replaced with a gurgling sound.

A jarring wakeup call jolts me upright. I say nothing to the woman and then drop the phone in the cradle with a crash. As always after this dream, I am panicked; heart racing, respirations pounding, sweat covering me. This nightmare is particularly disturbing, its relation to Billie obvious. I am not so sure I want to be here anymore. His death looms in my mind. The trapped expression on the man haunts me. The room seems small and I am claustrophobic.

I swing my legs over the edge of the bed, my head in my hands. My breathing slows. It is time. I grab my suitcase and find what I always want when this happens.

The bottle is reassuring. I caress it slowly, lovingly. Jim Beam, Sweet Amber; the finest Kentucky bourbon in my estimate, sits on the table before me. I remove the seal slowly and twist off the cap with deliberation. I swear I can smell the vintage aroma in the air. I have my favorite ground glass tumbler into which I pour two fingers worth. I sit and stare at the mixture. I worshiped that blend in the past. I am sweating again and a drop drips from my nose onto the round black Formica covered table. I pick up the glass in two hands which are trembling. With the glass at my lips, the smell is wonderful.

The knock on the door stops all that. I stand, check the window. Two officers are at the door. I recap the bottle, take it and my glass to the bathroom. I close the door behind me and move to the front door.

"Hello?" I stand at the door and realize that I am in my boxer shorts. I wipe the sweat from my brow.

"Hello, I am Captain Marvin Fulton of the TDCJ. How are you this morning Dr. Hickok?" Before me stands two gray uniformed officers in cowboy hats and black shiny boots. Marvin is a large, plump, black man with a short afro haircut, handcuffs, and an imposing looking holstered gun.

"I am fine." The guy does not know. I came so close to ruining 12 years of sobriety.

"I am here to escort you to the Walls Unit and Billie James Sampson. "

"Oh…". I look down at my outfit, boxer shorts, and wife beater shirt. "Well, that is nice. Can I get dressed?"

The trip to the Walls unit goes quickly. I follow the squad car in my Z. There is a patch of traffic at the light and Marvin flips on his lights and siren, skirting it. I follow through the light carefully. As we approach the prison I see the protestors again. There now are many lining both sides of 12th street. There are two opposing camps. On one side of the street, posters fly announcing the inhumanity of the death penalty. On the opposite side, the cruelty of the murderer is emphasized. The two groups seem to meet at the entrance gate to the prison.

We stop at the gate. Marvin gets out of the squad car.

"Move, yaw-all!" He puts one hand instinctively on his holstered gun and shoo's the sides apart. "Yaw-all move! Now! We're going through this gate."

One black-shirted man, a hangman's gallows stenciled on the front, with a wild afro haircut, stands at the center of the gate. "You're facilitating murder, Sir."

"I'll facilitate your arrest if yaw-all don't get moving!" Marvin grabs the man by the back of his shirt and hauls him aside. The gate opens remotely. He returns to the car. We drive slowly through the gate and into the Walls parking lot. I look over my shoulder. Afro-man is shaking his fist behind us.

I see now why it's called The Walls. A huge ancient, red-brick structure sits in front of me. It is several floors high, with tiny windows that look barred. There are turreted guard towers in each corner and brick steps that lead up to an imposing entrance.

The unit's nickname, of course, comes from the massive brick wall. Originally the walls were sandstone. In 1940, it was encased in the red bricks giving it its ominous appearance. The Texas prison system, always known for self-sufficiency, used bricks constructed by inmates.

We walk the long stairway to the entrance above, step after long step. As I trudge along, I see in my mind a chain-gang building the walls. They are dressed in starched white prison garb, with black numbers crudely stenciled on their backs. It is hot in the sweltering Texas sun. There are birds-of-prey circling above, tossing down caws of anguish. The men are chained together with several guards, complete with 12 gauge shotguns, cruelly overlooking them. One is quite close, and I see my reflection in his wire-rimmed sunglasses.

A man makes a move, running for his life. There are yells as the prisoners cheer him on. The guard with the sunglasses shoots the escaping inmate in the back, blood spurting. He writhes and falls to the ground on his face.

"You need to register in black ball-point pen. Please print and make it legible."

We are standing at a long counter now. A red-haired officer with a crooked smile hands me a brown wooden clipboard. The board has an attached chain and a masking taped black Bic ballpoint. The officer has a very distracting right facial twitch that makes him look like he is winking at me.

"You must write out your middle name."

I am Lee W. For so long, the name is one word to me. Yes, I do know what the W stands for but have not used that really ever. "It's W, Officer."

"You don't have a middle name?"

"Well yes, I do, but I don't use it."

"Well, today you use it. What does the W stand for?"

I reluctantly answer him. "Wiley."

"Well, then Wiley it is. Is that with one or two L's?" He stands ready to write in the name for me.

I grab the clipboard and print WILEY and hand it back to the man who smiles that crooked smile and twitches again. Marvin is standing next to me. He takes the clipboard from me and hands it to the officer. "Come with me, Hickok."

I next find myself in the warden's office. It is a large room with extensive cherry woodwork completing the walls, covered with books, a conference table, and the warden's desk. Windows look out on the yard below. I pull up a chair and sit in front of the desk.

Warden Charles Thomas O'Reilly is a tall thin man with a balding gray head and goatee beard. He wears round frameless glasses and has deep blue non-blinking eyes.

"So, Hickok…you want to view Sampson's event?"

The question seemed abrupt. I was here because Billie asked me. "I got a note in the mail asking me to come visit him. I suppose he wants me here when that happens. I don't know. Can I talk to him?"

"But you want to?"

"Want to what?"

"View the event?"

"I want to do whatever Billie wants me to do."

"How nice. Sampson has no friends or family. As of now, no one has arranged to be present. For some reason, he has chosen you to be the sole witness."

There was silence between us. I really did not know what to say.

"This is day 5, that is 5 days before the event. He is now out of death row, and in a holding cell next to the death chamber. There is a room where you can speak to him without encumbrances. Let me prepare you for this. Sampson is a violent murderer. He has been relatively well behaved on his tenure with us. Remember, however, that he is a vicious, malicious, brutal, killer, sexual deviant and assaulter. He will be shackled at all times. You can not touch him. You may spend one hour each day. Day 5 will be spent in the observation room, with no direct contact with the inmate. Do you have any questions?"

I thought but had no questions at that point. The Warden put his head down and began writing on a legal-size tablet of paper. He looked up surprised that I was still present. "You can go, Hickok!"

I found myself in a 12 by 12 room painted and covered in puke green linoleum. I sit in one of two chairs that face each other. Along the wall is an opaque window that I assume is one-way, with law enforcement on the other side. A second door to the right is visible. I wait some time, not knowing what to expect.

The door finally opens and through it walks Billie James Sampson. I remember him as a tallish man, but he has put on quite a bit of weight since his hospital days. He is dressed in a white cotton jumpsuit with the letters DR in black on the back. He is a light-skinned African-American with brilliant blue eyes. Two officers escort the shackled man into the room. He sits down, and they remove his arm shackles leaving his legs bound.

Billie smiles a big toothy smile. "Hi, Doc!"

Right up front, I realize that he has lost the gold-toothed smile. White teeth replace the gold-capped grill noted the last time I saw the man. The miracle of modern dental work in the Huntsville prison system is on display that day.

Chapter 22

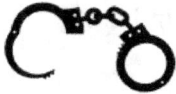

"Hi, Billie."

"Hi, Doc." Billie smiles. Again, I notice his dental work, an adequate job I think. Taxpayer's dollars, well spent. "How are you?"

Billie looks down at the floor and shakes his head affirmatively. There is a small smile on his face. "Fine, I mean okay, given the circumstances."

Right off I realize that Billie speaks very well. Eight years of time has improved this. No more I's this and I's that. No more fractured sentences. He uses complex words. He spoke as if he was educated. I wondered what he had done through these years to do so.

I had not come with an agenda or a list of questions. I wished I had, what do you say to a convicted murderer death row inmate who is on for execution? I decided to start with what caused me to meet the man, his urologic history. "I understand you still pass stones?"

"Ya, small ones. Usually, I feel this pressure right here." Billie lifted his jacket and wife-beater shirt and points to his right flank.

I notice the eagle tattoo on his chest and the well healed abdominal incision. "How often do yaw-all think you have a stone?"

Billie thinks and scratches his nearly shaven head. "Well, Doc, maybe every two weeks or so. I feel that feeling and then pass the stone into the toilet. I still have mucous. But…but the feeling is very mild, not even really a pain!"

"Good, that is what is supposed to happen. You drop a stone from your kidney and it travels in the ileal ureter. The ileum's diameter is large and so there is no obstruction and therefore no pain. Dr. Wilson says your kidney is working well. Great. Your operation is a success!" There is a sly smile on Billie's face. I think he is wondering why it is a success when this week he will be executed. I just shake my head in agreement. It is an ironic twist for sure.

Billie chuckles quietly. "It has been nice these last years, though. I really have no kidney stone pain like before. I have passed a stone every week or so since I was a kid. Pain made me mean, Doc." Billie looked down. He thought and responded. "I made me mean, Doc. Always was mean. As long as I can remember I was mean as heck. You know fights, stealing and such."

"Tell me about that Billie. I mean the crime and such, what happened to you?"

Billie rubbed his face. He looked at the guard. "Can I take this jacket off Boss? Really hot in here!" The guard indicated that he could, and Billie set the white cotton jacket down on the floor next to him. He took a small black bible out of the pocket and set it on his thigh. By choice, the TDCJ kept the temperature at 85 degrees. I agreed I was hot as well, beginning to sweat.

"I grew up in Lubbock. My mother was a whore, never really saw her. Don't really remember her. She died real young. An O/D I think. My Daddy beat the heck out of me all the time. Did more than that too." He left it at that and looked down at the floor.

I remembered the dossier. "Did he rape you?"

There is a long pause. Billie moves his bible to the other thigh. "Sure enough did, all the time in fact." He looks down.

There is an obvious sadness in the man. "I beat him up though, last time I ever saw him. I guess I got him." He looks up at me. Seems to be looking for some acceptance.

I recalled the baseball bat. The *weapon of choice* the dossier said. It's brutality returns to my mind. The autopsy pictures flash in my mind. I wonder how much he wants to talk? I decide to try something very uncomfortable. "Do you think about her? Ya know, the dead girl?" I guess that he will walk out on me, but he doesn't.

Billie moves the bible again. He looks down and rubs his head. "I do…all the time. She didn't deserve what I did, Doc. Rita Maxwell." He looks up, his blue eyes piercing me. "That was her name, Doc. Pretty girl. I knew her from before. Picked her up at Thirsty Thirties. Raped her and beat her to death. Knew that I would the moment I saw her in the bar. They say I ran over her hand. She had a wedding ring on." Billie shakes his head, negatively, firmly. This seems important to him. "That's messed up. Didn't know that!"

Billie looks at me again. I sense that he is looking to me for some forgiveness. How can I; I wonder? I didn't know the girl of course. But the brutality, the autopsy pictures leave me so uncomfortable. I am just silent.

"She was just a bartender. Just a simple girl, a real sweetheart. Understand she had a little girl as well. Guess I ruined that girl's life, too. Wish I could do it over, but I can't. Going to pay for it, just 5 days, Doc."

I let the last statement hang in the air. There was silence and then I asked. "Have you ever killed anyone else," I wonder? I keep thinking he will walk out on me, but he doesn't. He's uncomfortable, however.

Billie looks down. There is a long pause. He looks at the guard. "Ya beat a man in a bar. Never got beat down for that. Don't know why. Guess the guy had it coming to him or something. I beat many people, hurt many people, Doc."

"Why did you ask me to visit you, Billie?"

Billie is obviously troubled by this question. "I know it's tough, Doc. I figured you'd come. That time in Galveston was the happiest time in my life."

I am very surprised at this. "Why's that?"

"Yaw-all cared for me. Yaw-all tried to help me. Also, of course, I found the Lord." With this, there is a big smile on his face. He picks up his Bible and holds it out in front of him. It is a small, oldish looking black bible with tattered pages. I can tell that it is his prized possession. He beams as he opens it.

"I have a verse for you, Doc!" Billie looks to me for acknowledgment as he opens the bible flipping expertly through the text.

I shake my head yes and sit back in my chair.

"It is from the New Testament. First Corinthians ten thirteen."

"…who will not suffer you to be tempted above that your able…"

"Do you know what that means Doc?"

I am a believer and at one time a Born-Again Christian. I have to say, however, that right now I did not see the connection. Billie is excited. "No, I am not really sure, Billie."

"It applies to your visit here Doc. You see, God gives us tasks, but he won't give us one beyond our abilities. You're here this week for a purpose Doc. Just have faith that you're helping. You are Doc, helping me greatly."

I am touched by his sincerity. Billie loves the bible. Wouldn't it be wonderful if he could stay at Huntsville and preach? What a waste. "Do you have a favorite verse?"

Billie chuckles quietly. He has lit up now, and he flips through the bible.

"It is so obvious Doc! It is from the New Testament again. John fourteen six."

> *"I am the way the truth and the life. No one comes to the Father except through me."*

"Are you a believer Doc?"

Billie closes his Bible and again puts it gently on his knee. He is so alive at this moment. He looks to me with an air of hopeful light. Now my salvation is a complicated question. Yes, I am a believer. I was saved years ago but have fallen away from the practice. I believe that Jesus Christ is Lord and Savior and that salvation is only possible through him. At that moment, it is so ironic, I want to feel the faith that Billie feels. "I am a believer Billie, but I am really lost right now!"

"Are you familiar with John sixteen thirty-three?"

Right now, I couldn't quote Genesis one verse one. "Not at this moment Billie. Read it to me!"

"In the world, you will have tribulation. But take heart I have overcome the world!"

"Don't you see Doc? Coming here is your tribulation. Or let's just say it is a tribulation in your life. You just need to have faith that you can get through it with dignity, and comfort this murdering sinner. You are Doc. You are helping me so much. You know that no one else is coming?" Billie looked down. He cried a few tears and wiped them with the back of his hand. "After all these years I have no one, but you came, and I, and God as well, am so grateful. "

I wished at that time that I could hug Billie. He needed it and so did I. I looked at the guard who just shook his head no.

There was a pause here. I thought about my next question. Thought I would ask a non-threatening one. "Billie, you speak and read so well. How did you get educated?"

Billie laughs. "Well, yaw-all remember my reading in Galveston?"

I shake my head yes. I recall him reading *The Cat in the Hat* at the hospital. "What was that woman's name that helped you?"

"Mrs. Carol Winegarten," he says really quickly as if she is a prominent figure in his life. "She was real nice. Got me interested in reading. She really started me thinking I could get educated, Doc. I wasn't much in school. You know, dropped out and all. So, I got my GED. And then I took some correspondence courses and got an AA degree. Just in general ED. So, there I am, Doc. But the Bible, now that's what I really got learned on. It's my thing." Here he picks up the tattered Bible and points it at me. "Doc, I want you to have this, you know after I'm gone. Really the only thing I own, so would you take it?"

I am touched. I find myself almost crying. "I would be honored," I say after consoling myself. I decide to touch another sad subject. "How do you want to be buried, Billie?"

Billie surprises me. He smiles the biggest smile. "Could I be buried in Galveston, Doc? You know, it is real nice down there. The Gulf and all. You think they would allow that?"

I think in my mind. I decide to facilitate that. I will take care of all the arrangements and costs. "Yes, Billie. I will make sure of it. There is a real nice cemetery near the beach. Would you like that?"

Billie just smiles. He shakes his head yes. "Say, I really hurt that chief. You know, Dr. Dana. I roughed her up just awful. Will you make sure she knows that I am so sorry?"

"I will specifically talk to her, Billie. I will tell her that we had this discussion. She will forgive you. I know her."

"That's one-hour Dr. Hickok." The guard is standing by Billie. He puts handcuffs on his wrists. He takes Billie away through the side door. I stand and move behind him. "I will see you Billie, tomorrow."

Billie looks over his shoulder as he is led away. "Wouldn't miss it for the world, Doc."

Chapter 23

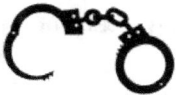

The days rolled by quickly, one eventful day after another. My one hour each morning was spent talking about a wide variety of subjects. I really enjoyed what Billie had become. To think that his execution was so close was heartbreaking. I believed I had a purpose in being here, however. I did become, as the days moved on, more comfortable with my task. I began to sleep better, no further dreams, and I did not resort to Sweet Amber. Tragically, days four through two were over before I knew it.

    We talked about his lawyers and appeals. It seemed as if he had many attorneys, all trying to get him to appeal the conviction and sentence. He was a poor illiterate Texas minority, and there were many grounds for appeal that the councilors pushed. From the very beginning, he waved all of this. It was difficult, however; he was expected to fight for his life. Billie wanted to live but he really wanted to live in heaven. He also felt he deserved to die. It is odd, but this convicted murderer was a conservative person through and through. He believed in capital punishment and the ultimate retribution. He believed in its good to society. He believed that he was guilty of first-degree murder and deserved to be executed by the state. So, after proving his mental competency, he was able to wave further appeals. The result was that his execution date became closer and closer.

I was fascinated by what life on death row was like. The Death Row inmate spends almost his entire time alone in a 60-square-foot cell. The cells have a small window at one end. The steel door has a narrow slot and, at the bottom, a slit through which guards slide food trays. Basically, only sound penetrates these cement boxes. Prison is a loud place and sound can cause the most torment. Taunting, clanging doors, and yelling never ceases. There are dull thuds of beatings and screaming. Billie was a lucky one, he possessed a set of foam rubber ear plugs which he used continuously.

When they do get out for exercise for some short time five days a week, they can only exercise alone in adjacent cages. Contact visits and televisions are never allowed in what is perhaps the harshest death row conditions in the country.

In Billie's cell, there was no television, something I always thought prisoners had. He possessed a small transistor radio that got broken reception only when he was able to afford a battery. Billie owned two books. The Bible he so loved was given to him by the prison chaplain. In addition, he owned a tattered copy of *My Utmost for His Highest by Oswald Chambers, the devotional that he read every morning. He received this through the mail, through a church outreach program by Billy Graham. His reading came from the prison library where he was allowed only one book a month. He was able through the years to read numerous books and eventually acquire his AA degree. He read all the great classics, where A Tale of Two Cities and War and Peace were especially enjoyed. In the former, he loved* Madame Defarge the revenge-minded villainess who is continually knitting. In the latter, he loved Prince Andrei Nikolayevich Bolkonsky hero of the Napoleonic war.

The Warden, Charles Marcy Thomas rules over the prison with an iron hand. He has overseen more executions, 101, than any individual in US history. He was fine with Billie's decision to stop appeals. "Too many damn appeals in this world." He was quoted as saying in a 1976 piece in Rolling Stone. It is creepy, but he will be the last voice that Billie will hear in this world. Needless to say, his is not a comforting voice.

The guards vary in their humanity. Some like Captain Marvin Fulton are dedicated public servants and equally fine human beings. He was the ward captain during most of Billie's stay, and Billie has nothing but nice words for the man. Some like officer Drew Kinsky, are sadistic bastards. The man would turn on ice cold water whenever Billie's rare showers were ongoing. He would often forget Billie's meager meal and bring it at the end of the shift cold. Yes, prison life was something that you would rather forget.

The food was the one thing in a prisoner's life that they look forward to. In Huntsville, that food was a product of a chef named Antonio Gonzales. He was a huge plump man dressed in white cotton clothes. He constantly wore a white headband over his balding head and sweated continually in the 85-degree environment. He was charged with creating some 750 gallons of food each day. In doing so he shone as a true chef and cared about his food. And so, there were Monday pizza, Tuesday burger, Wednesday pork chop,

Thursday spaghetti, Friday corn fritters, Saturday omelet, and Sunday chicken fried steak. Billie enjoyed these meals as long as Drew Kinsky wasn't staffing his ward.

Day two began with our usual salutation.

"Hi, Billie."

"Hi, Doc."

"Are you sleeping well?" My sleeping had smoothed out and I wondered how a man so close to execution was doing.

"Not really sleeping Doc. Too many thoughts in my head. When I do sleep my dreams are so brutal." He tells me about one of his dreams. "I have my baseball bat and I am alone on a dark street corner. I have to defend myself from a group of boys, but I really don't want to hurt anyone."

I imagine the dream is disconcerting. It is a sign of his recovery I think, his violent history a thing of the past. I try to put myself in Billie's place. The fright of each passing day must be overwhelming.

I understand that Billie gets a last meal request. "What are you requesting for your last meal?"

Billie looks down. He obviously has given this a lot of thought. "I would order a sirloin steak, but they won't bring that. They'll bring a ground beef steak instead. So, I am going to have a double hamburger with thick slabs of cheddar cheese, mustard, catchup, mayo, and fresh juicy onions. I am going to request fries, a huge pile smothered in chili. On the side, I want grits and fried okra. Then to top it off I want a piece of peach pie. I would get a scoop of vanilla ice cream, but it would just melt in this heat. I won't be able to eat it all probably. Maybe won't be able to eat at all. You know, I want to go, you know peace in God's presence, but I am scared Doc." Billie looked at me, his blue eyes sympathetic.

"Billie, I can imagine. I have a Bible verse for you." I felt joy in my heart. I had taken the *Gideons* Bible at the motel that night and perused it. It took a while, but I got a feel for the Bible back and that was peaceful. "It is from John 14:2." Billie repeated the verse with me from memory.

"My Father's house has many rooms; if that were not so, would I have told you that I am going there to prepare a place for you?"

The verse to me is awe-inspiring. I imagined a white, golden floored mansion trimmed in pearl. Floating in the air, it is filled with angelic beings. Within is flowing sparkling water and a fresh perfumed aroma. Each *guest* gets a room complete with a white scented bed and vases of lavender lilacs.

"Must be nice." Billie is in a peaceful place. He has closed his eyes and smiling a big smile. "Doc, I can see it. Each room is so quiet and beautiful. There are angels at the doors. Music plays quietly. In some ways Doc, I can hardly wait. What a great God to accept me." He opens his eyes. "I am the world's greatest sinner, Doc. The things I have done. How can He forgive someone like me?"

"I guess that is what God's all about, Billie."

Chapter 24

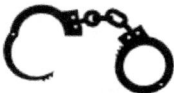

The day of execution arrived on a stormy central Texas day. It was scheduled for the stroke of midnight, April 23, 1993. I arrived early that morning. I had petitioned to spend more than an hour with Billie that day. When I walked into the prison in the morning, I expected my request to be denied. Captain Marvin Fulton met me at the reception area.

"How yaw-all this morning, Dr. Hickok?"

"Well, I could be better." I looked at the Captain. We both nodded, understanding that this was the last day of Billie James Sampson's short stint on earth. "What did the warden decide?"

"Well, he has a proposition for you."

I looked at the man with a question. "What does he have in mind?"

"Well, if yaw-all will meet with the press concerning your time with the prisoner, and if that press release is acceptable to the warden, you can stay. All day if you want and be here at midnight. If that's what you want, Dr. Hickok."

"Yaw-all are kidding. Is that it?"

"That's it. But let me warn you."

I thought he was going to warn me of an antagonistic press, an experience with rabid reporters who vehemently opposed capital punishment. I imagined a room filled with the media, cameras, and microphones. "Warn me about what?"

The captain looked uncomfortable. He took his hat off and wiped his brown. "You aren't going to like it."

"Like what," I wondered?

What he said turned out to be kind. He was warning me about an event that would leave such a lasting impression on me. "This event, the execution. It isn't very pleasant Dr. Hickok!"

I had an idea about that. I never, however, thought that it would be so weighty. Well, I never thought it would be pleasant. I have to stay. The man has no one. "I don't really owe him, but you know after this week I kind of owe him."

"It is up to yaw-all. Think about it seriously though Dr. Hickok. Think about what you're going to witness."

"Point taken, Captain."

The Captain led me through a long hallway and to a door labeled *Press*. I found myself again thinking of what I would find with *the Press*. The image of CNN reporters crowded around an astronaut leaving for the moon flashed in my brain. They were fighting to get their questions answered, pushing against the man. Microphones were forced into the man's face. I took a deep breath and opened the door.

Inside sat a single man at a table. He was a young longish brown-haired man who tied his do into a short ponytail. He had intense brown eyes and a poorly groomed beard. He was dressed in a grey ratty Houston Astro's Tee-shirt, brown corduroy pants, and Birkenstocks. He stood up when I approached him. "Dr. Hickok; Dr. Lee W. Hickok?"

"Yes, that is me." I was a little disappointed. Always the showman, I sort of hoped for a room full of a bevy of reporters.

He reached and shook my hand. "I am Monty Walker from KRDK. I am here to get a press release concerning your time with Billie James Sampson. Sit here," he said directing me to a chair on the opposite side of the table. Between us was a microphone connected to a small tape recorder that looked to be held together with masking tape. "State your full name and place of residence into the recorder."

"Lee W. Hickok, University of Texas Medical Branch, Department of Urology, Galveston, Texas."

"Dr. Hickok what relation have you had with the inmate BSJ?"

"He is my patient and recently I have become a spiritual advisor to the man."

"How long have you known BSJ?"

"I first met him in 1985 at UTMB. We eventually operated on him."

"What would you say is your role in the events of today?"

"I am an advisor, a friend, and colleague."

"State for us your impression of the prison staff."

Here I realized that the warden would be especially concerned about my answer. "I have been impressed with the dedication and competence of the TDCJ staff. At all points, they have been humane, efficient, and professional. All in all, considering the event's magnitude, my experience with the TDCJ has been excellent."

"Okay, anything else you need to add?"

I thought about this question. "I want to thank warden Thomas for his hospitality. Nothing further."

They moved our visiting room for the last day. It was a bigger room with chairs lined up around the periphery. It was for a larger audience in the waning hours before an execution. Sadly, Billie did not have a crowd. Billie was sitting in one chair when I entered. Gone were the shackles. Billie stood up with a smile on his face. He crossed the room to meet me, and we embraced for the first time.

I looked at the man in the face. He looked tired, bloodshot eyes. "Did you sleep, Billie?"

Billie sat down slowly. "No, Doc. Didn't sleep a wink last night. I am excited, sort of. Really looking forward to getting off this planet. But I kept going over and over all those that I hurt. One time I robbed an 80-year-old vet. I'll never forget him. Walked with a cane. I broke into his house at night. Had a gun and praise the Lord didn't kill him. The old guy woke up. I had a tip about a stash of bills in his bookcase. The guy begged me not to take it. Cried, Doc he actually cried and told me he was saving to help his son with his battle with cancer." Billie looked down. He shook his head sadly. "You know I beat the guy up and took all his money. As I left I grabbed a chicken leg that was in the refrigerator. I am bad, Doc. Really deserve my punishment. I could tell yaw-all so many stories like that."

"Does Sara Shagshaw have any kin? You know, anyone you could apologize to?"

"I wrote her daughter a letter, Doc. Leslie was her name. About 16 now. Really laid it on the line. Told her how sorry I was. Got a letter back from the girl. Told me to rot in Hell. She said she was looking forward to seeing me get the needle. Doc, I don't blame her. Took her Mother away. So brutal. How could I do that?"

"Were you high on drugs, Billie?"

"Oh, yea. I was into meth at that time. Used a rock just before I went into the bar. But Doc, that's not an excuse. I'm bad, that's it." He looked down dejectedly. He reached for his Bible and flipped through the pages.

"Romans 3:23 says: "for all have sinned and fall short of the glory of God." You know, praise God for his grace. I need it more than anyone. If it wasn't for this Bible, I don't know would have probably hung myself in my cell."

I decided at that moment to open up to the man. Until this time, I was very impersonal with my life, not sharing much of importance. "Billie, I will tell you a story. I am an alcoholic. Big time drinker. Used to drink when I was operating."

"Were yaw-all drinking when you operated on me?"

I thought back in my mind. "No, and this is true. I quit drinking years before." I actually had to concentrate on the years involved. "No that was 85 when we operated on you. I quit drinking in 81. What I wanted to tell you is how I quit drinking. Now I drank every day, all day long. Like I said I drank in the operating room. My drink of choice was Kentucky bourbon, you know Sweet Amber." I pictured in my mind my bottle at the motel. I had a desire to drink again. "I decided to quit. Drank up all the booze in my house. I remember sitting naked with my red, white, and blue, USA cowboy boots in my bathtub drinking beer, bourbon and whatever else I had in my house. Was drunk beyond imagination. Then I stopped and went to sleep. When I woke up I was hallucinating. Had a real case of DT's. Started an IV in my own arm and medicated myself until I woke up. Amber. My wife is named Amber. She's a nurse. And she was there to comfort me. Now that's an alcoholic, my friend. And God has forgiven me!"

"I know you have done such bad things, Billie. I know that, and you're going to get your punishment. But there are many bad people in this world. The deal is that God forgives you. It is amazing really."

There was a knock on the door. It opens and in walks the Chaplain. He is dressed in black clothes with a white collar. Gary Nelson is a tall, good-looking man with intense blue eyes. Billie knows the man. They embrace. Billie shows him the signature page of his Bible. It is addressed to Billie signed by the Chaplain. Billie and the Chaplain sit down and encourage me to sit with them. I wonder whether the two should be alone.

"Doc, sit here next to me," Billie says.

He gestures to me. I pull up a chair and sit. Billie wonders about the Chaplain's family. They are fine, but the Chaplain is here for Billie.

"How are you, Billie?"

"It's tough Chaplain. Not sleeping well. Having dreams. Really want to get this over. The Doc has helped me, though." Billie puts his arm around my shoulder. He is sincere, and I finally realize that my trip was worth all the trouble.

"I want to read from the Bible, Billie. I want to read about the Garden of Gethsemane, from Matthew 26: verses 36 to 46. Billie will read the first verses, 36 to 38. Then I'll read verses 39 through 42. After that Doc, you finish up with verses 42 through 46."

Billie took his bible and expertly flips to the passage.

[36] Then Jesus went with his disciples to a place called Gethsemane, and he said to them, "Sit here while I go over there and pray." [37] He took Peter and the two sons of Zebedee along with him, and he began to be sorrowful and troubled. [38] Then he said to them, "My

soul is overwhelmed with sorrow to the point of death. Stay here and keep watch with me."

"This passage is relevant, Billie and Doc. Jesus knows that he will be executed. He has great sorrow. Peter, John, and James are with him as he prays. The Chaplain opens his Bible. He, like Billie, is an expert and he flips to the verses in Matthew.

[39] Going a little farther, he fell with his face to the ground and prayed, "My Father, if it is possible, may this cup be taken from me. Yet not as I will, but as you will."

[40] Then he returned to his disciples and found them sleeping. "Couldn't you men keep watch with me for one hour?" he asked Peter. [41] "Watch and pray so that you will not fall into temptation. The spirit is willing, but the flesh is weak."

[42] He went away a second time and prayed, "My Father, if it is not possible for this cup to be taken away unless I drink it, may your will be done."

"The men are weak Billie and Doc. The can't stay awake and pray with him. Jesus is not disappointed I would say. He knows the weakness of the flesh"

Billie hands me his bible. It is open to the verse. I read:

[43] When he came back, he again found them sleeping, because their eyes were heavy. [44] So he left them and went away once more and prayed the third time, saying the same thing.

[45] Then he returned to the disciples and said to them, "Are you still sleeping and resting? Look, the hour has come, and the Son of Man

is delivered into the hands of sinners. [46] Rise! Let us go! Here comes my betrayer!"

We all three sit and ponder what we have read. Billie speaks first. "Chaplain, thank you for that. I am not Jesus though. He suffered for all of mankind. He was betrayed by Judas, the Devil. I can relate to him so much, however."

The door opens and in walks Captain Fulton and his entourage. I look at the clock, it's twenty minutes to midnight.

"It's time, Billie." The men shackle Billie quickly. I wonder whether that is necessary at this point, but that's the state of Texas.

Billie turns to me. "Here Doc. Where I am going I won't need it." Billie hands me his old Bible. I tear up and embrace the man. The group leads Billie away.

Captain Fulton stays behind. "Are you two staying for the event?"

Event, there is that word again. It was used by the warden and the officers as well. *It's an execution!* I want to yell. The chaplain looks at me. "Yes, I am staying until the end!"

Chapter 25

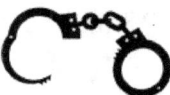

The Allan B. Polunsky death chamber at the Walls unit in Huntsville, Texas consists of a small soundproofed room built with cement cinder blocks and painted a calm turquoise green. At the center of the room sits the gurney, stocked with cotton white padding and two arm boards with brown leather restraints. To its left, a slanted mirror is mounted that allows the executioner to see the inmate during the procedure. A small slot sits below the mirror, allowing the entry of tubing used for delivering the lethal potion. To the right of the gurney is a large curtained window which covers the viewing area, split into two separate rooms for the prisoner's family and the victim's family.

    Lethal injection involves the establishment of an intravenous line through which is introduced a three-drug combination. The first drug is sodium thiopental, infused as an anesthetic to put the inmate into a deep sleep. Pancuronium bromide follows to paralyze the prisoner. The last drug is potassium chloride which stops the heart and causes death.

The Chaplain and I are led to the viewing room. Within are chairs lined up in six empty rows which face a large royal blue curtain across the front.

I think we both are in shock of sorts. Neither of us knows what to say. We both sit down in the front row.
"Have you ever done this before, Chaplain?" I am nervous now and look at my watch which says 11:45 pm. The room is small, and I am claustrophobic. Someone must have turned up the heat, for I find myself sweating. I am sick to my stomach. I hope that I will not vomit.

The Chaplain looks at me. He is nervous as well, I am sure. He seems to be sweating, drops on his brow. He looks down at the floor. "This is my second execution I am afraid, Lee W. The first was Howard Marcus Washington. They worked for one hour trying to get an IV in. He died crying. Struggling as well. He was yelling and kicking. It was gruesome, I hope it goes better for Billie."

I tried to divert my thoughts. I thought in my mind starting IV's in difficult subjects. Billie is thin, the obese especially hard candidates. I am not sure about Billie's drug use history. He mentioned methamphetamine used before the murder. IV drug use is definitely a risk factor for difficult access. I am so glad that it is not me starting the line.

My mind returns to the physician who will pronounce Billie's death. I recall as a newbie intern having to do this on an ancient old man in the VA hospital. Nurse *Ratched* had told me that the man was dead. "Get in there and pronounce him." At that point in my training, I really didn't know what to do. I entered a darkened room anxiously; very nervous. I find a frail gray-haired man with closed eyes lying alone in a hospital bed. There were wilted lilacs in a vase I remember. He looked dead. I stood at the foot of his bed for the longest time. He seemed to not be breathing. I took my stethoscope and listened for breath sounds and then for a heartbeat. Much to my surprise, there were signs of life. To my horror, the man sat up with a bolt and opened his eyes yelling: "I am not dead yet you little crapper!"

"I am sure glad I'm not starting his IV!"

Overhead I notice something that I found as odd. Playing quietly was piped in music. The tune was *Whiskey Lullaby,* I think by Garth Brooks. I thought about Sweet Amber and wished I had a shot right now.

The curtain opens slowly. A spotlight flashes on. Within the death chamber lays Billie. He is on the gurney, his arms strapped to the arm boards. There is an IV in his right arm hooked to tubing that exits through the slot in the wall. With him stands a male nurse. A man in a gray suit stands by his side.

The nurse raises the head of the gurney so that he can be seen. He has some trouble doing this. Billie is jolted to the position. He is ashen and pallid, his blue eyes closed. He is mumbling to himself. Knowing him I know he is praying to God.

The man in the suit reads from a document. "William James Sampson, you are hereby condemned to death by lethal injection by the great state of Texas for the crime of first-degree murder." I can hear crying coming from the room next door. Someone yells: "murderer!"

"Do you have any last words, William James Sampson?" The man in the suit turns to Billie. He places the document in his coat pocket. He is tapping his cowboy-booted foot for some strange reason.

Billie's eyes open. He looks at the man and then into the room alongside us. "Yes, I do." He clears his throat and speaks. "I am guilty of a… awful murder, death… I accept my punishment. To the Maxwell family and…and especially Leslie, I am…" At this point, he seems to cry. The man in the suit takes a handkerchief from his pocket and wipes his eyes. Billie takes several deep breaths and continues. "I am very sorry for taking your Rita…and Mother from you. Especially like that. It was a brutal act, and I hope that my death helps you…some, anyway. I am a sinner and an evil man." Billie coughs, swallows and continues. "I have been saved by Jesus Christ…the Savior of the world."

With that Billie turns his head and looks at the man in the suit. He nods and says: "Sir I am ready."

The man opens a stop-cock on the IV tubing. Billie's eyes close. He takes a deep breath and then there is nothing.

Chapter 26

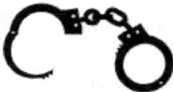

Lenny Kravitz, *Fly Away,* blasts from my radio as I fly in my 240 Z over the Galveston Causeway. The Causeway carries traffic over Galveston Bay and the Gulf Intracoastal Waterway. It is the main access to Galveston Island. It is a beautiful spring day, April 25, 1993. The sun is setting over the gulf, billowing clouds cover the blue sky, and seabirds are flying high in the air. I drive with the windows down and the radio set to a blasting volume. I am so glad to return to Galveston. The execution of Billie James Sampson is something I will never forget. I have seen things and learned others that will be etched in my mind forever. Billie turned out to be a great friend. His death was sad, but his life was uplifting, at least his spiritual growth at the end.

His death in some way revitalized my faith. I am excited about this New Life. I plan to live accordingly, practicing what

Jesus said in Matthew 6:33: "But seek first the kingdom of God then all these things will be given to you."

His bible sits on the passenger seat along with some of his sparse possessions. Billie wrote me a short note that I found in its pages. "Dear Brother," it read again written in blue crayon. "When you get this, I will be gone from this life and in paradise. Be happy for me, I am free! Thank you, Lee W., for your friendship and fellowship before my death. I know that you suffered for me and I appreciate it. In 2 Timothy 4:7 Paul says: *I have fought the good fight. I have finished the race. I have kept the faith.* I am not the apostle Paul, but I feel this verse applies in some small way to my life.

The Causeway becomes Broadway and I turn west on 61st street going towards the sea. Lakeview Cemetery sits overlooking the gulf. Beautiful green grass, lined by rows of brilliant white headstones, outline the beautiful seacoast. I find Billie's intended grave site. It has been prepared for his burial next week. I find myself tearing up. How dare I, I realize. Billie is in paradise.

www.ingramcontent.com/pod-product-compliance
Lightning Source LLC
Chambersburg PA
CBHW052147220526
45471CB00004B/1565